W9-BNA-211

# Aromatherapy Blends and Remedies

Over 800 recipes for everyday use

◆ ◇ ◆ ◇ ◆ ◇ ◆ ◇ ◆ ◇ ◆ ◇ ◆ ◇ ◆ ◇ ◆ ◇ ◆ ◇ ◆ ◇ ◆ ◇ ◆ ◇ ◆ ◇ ◆ ◇ ◆ ◇ ◆ ◇ ◆ ◇ ◆ ◇

## Franzesca Watson

*Illustrated by Christine Lane*

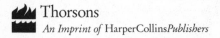
Thorsons
*An Imprint of* HarperCollins*Publishers*

Thorsons
An Imprint of HarperCollins*Publishers*
77–85 Fulham Palace Road,
Hammersmith, London W6 8JB
1160 Battery Street,
San Francisco, California 94111–1213

Published by Thorsons 1995
10  9  8  7  6  5

© Franzesca Watson 1995
© Illustrations by Christine Lane 1995

Franzesca Watson asserts the moral right to
be identified as the author of this work

A catalogue record for this book
is available from the British Library

ISBN 0 7225 3222 9

Printed in Great Britain by
Woolnough Bookbinding Ltd.,
Irthlingborough, Northants

All rights reserved. No part of this publication may be
reproduced, stored in a retrieval system, or transmitted,
in any form or by any means, electronic, mechanical,
photocopying, recording or otherwise, without the prior
permission of the publishers.

# Aromatherapy Blends and Remedies

There is a remedy for every illness
to be found in nature.

*Hippocrates (460–377 BC)*

Other titles in the Thorsons Aromatherapy series:

*Aromatherapy Massage*
*Aromatherapy for Lovers*
*Aromatherapy and the Mind*
*Aromatherapy for Women*
*Aromatherapy Workbook*
*Creative Aromatherapy*
*The Fragrant Year*
*Practical Aromatherapy*

By the same author:

*Aromatherapy for You at Home* (Natural by Nature Oils Ltd, 1991, 1994)

About the author:

Franzesca Watson is founder and managing director of Natural by Nature Oils Ltd, which selects and supplies aromatherapy oils throughout the UK and overseas. The company is based in London and has been established since 1974. She is also founder and principal of the International School of Aromatherapy.

To My Dear Mother,
**Despina**
the most special person in my life,
who inspired in me a fascination
for herbs and essential oils.

*Note to the Reader:*

This book was written to help the reader with everyday common conditions. It is not intended as a medical textbook. In cases of serious conditions the help of a doctor should be sought. It is always advisable to read the instructions carefully before using essential oils.

# Contents

# ◆ Introduction

My introduction to herbal remedies and essential oils began with my mother. I remember her telling us about her childhood in the town of Korthi on the island of Andros in Greece, where natural herbs remained popular long after they fell out of favour in Britain. At that time there were no conventional doctors or hospitals where she lived. It was not until she was about 18 years of age and went to a hospital in Athens to have her tonsils removed that she was first treated by a doctor. It was there that she met my father, who is English, as he was in the army and stationed in Athens.

The local people on my mother's island depended on what were called 'herb doctors' for their health care. In their own community they were completely self-sufficient. Recipes were handed down from generation to generation for various cures. My mother learned from her mother, who knew a great deal about using herbs and oils. They used to collect almonds and olives to press to make their own oils and various domestic remedies.

On my frequent visits to Greece as a young girl I used to help my aunts collect the herbs and beat the fruits off the trees to take home for pressing. Some of my intuitive ideas about the benefits of essential oils were formed as a result of my early experiences in Korthi. When I visited many years later, it was amazing to see how my relatives have kept to the old ways of collecting wild herbs and making their own natural remedies. There are many members of my mother's family still living an old-fashioned way of life in a very rural part of the island.

Within a year of meeting my parents were married, and then I was born, followed by my brother and sister one and two years later. We were brought up in a small village in Hampshire. Even then my mother used to take us early in the morning to collect herbs down Winkleberry Lane. She taught us how to select the useful herbs and avoid the poisonous plants. Although my mother had gathered only wild herbs when she was in rural Greece, she grew her own herbs when she came to live in England with my father.

I very much cherish my childhood memories of the Hampshire fields, the wonderful jars of herbs and the aroma of dried flowers hanging in different parts of the house.

Whenever any of us picked up a childhood illness we were treated with only natural remedies. The herb which always comes to my mind is the chamomile flower, which my mother would boil up and use for treating all sorts of infections. It is remarkable that I never went for any conventional treatment until I had to have my tonsils taken out, just as my mother had all those years ago.

When I had my own children I continued to use herbs and oils for their childhood illnesses. Except for some minor surgery, my whole family have depended only on natural remedies.

One year, just prior to Christmas, my elder son Simon ate some wild berries while on a survival trip in Canada, and developed such a severe rash all over his body that he was told he would probably not be allowed to travel on the plane home. He telephoned me for one of my remedies. I immediately mixed a selection of essential oils in a cream and promptly dispatched it to him. Thankfully, this cleared up his problem in time to enable him to make it home for the family's festive dinner.

Throughout the years when I was raising my children I developed many more recipes, adding to those I had learned from my mother. It was also during this time that my interest in massage developed, as massage complements essential oils perfectly. This led to the setting up of my own clinic.

I am sure my career in aromatherapy would not have happened and this book would not have been written without my mother's early influence on me. She passed on to me her fascination and respect for nature's herbs and their essential oils. My own two sons have also taken to the family tradition. A peek into their cupboards at any time will reveal a range of little bottles of essential oils.

As a professional therapist, I spend so much time advising other people that I hardly have time to look after myself. However, I must confess to having a weakness for a foot massage using my three favourite oils: frankincense, rose and neroli. Trust me to choose the most expensive ones!

Having spent my entire life involved with essential oils, my enthusiasm has continued to grow and I now wish to share with you all the many recipes I have created over the years.

In the writing of this book I have had to recall much from the last 25 years. At times it has been very exhausting, but I feel a sense of pride and fulfilment now that the book is finally completed. I have benefited directly from essential oils at all stages of my life, and never more so than during the many evenings I spent 'burning the midnight oils' writing this book. These oils have been a great comfort and inspiration to me. Many of the recipes in this book were written during my travels to different parts of the world. Appropriately enough, the section on holidays and first-aid was written while I was visiting the Florida Keys.

Now established as the fastest growing form of natural healing, aromatherapy is attracting powerful media attention and becoming highly popular. With so many books on aromatherapy already on the market, it was my intention to produce a book with easy-to-follow instructions and useful recipes so that readers can adopt a holistic approach to health, using essential oils for their physical, mental and emotional well-being.

We should stop relying so much on doctors and the over-burdened health service for our common everyday ailments, and instead use the natural home remedies that have been proven through the centuries and are so widely available.

The emphasis of this book is on recipes which call for only commercially available essential oils, so that you can easily buy them from your local health food shop and other outlets. Some readers may doubt the effects of essential oils. I can only say that, judging from my own experience and that of my regular clients, essential oils work. However, it takes a lot of practice to be able to blend the correct essential oils for a particular condition while at the same time achieving a balanced blend. The recipes in this book have been tried and tested and provide you with a short cut to using the oils with confidence.

My expertise is in blending, as I have a natural skill for being able to tell instantly if a blend is right or wrong before mixing. It is this knowledge that I am passing on to you.

It is my wish that this book will add to the current knowledge of essential oils and play a significant role in the development of aromatherapy. There is much we can learn from the simple plants gracing our earth; my fondest hope is that after reading this book you will have a better appreciation of the wonderful world of natural fragrance. As the most concentrated form of herbal healing, these beautiful essential oils are a gift to us from nature. Let their indisputable benefits be a part of your life.

*Personal Note:*

I must mention that I totally deplore cruelty to animals of any description. Since my early twenties I have been a strict vegetarian and I do not believe that the killing of animals for human consumption is either necessary or justifiable. The way animals are treated these days is absolutely barbaric. As a member of the Cosmetics Industry Coalition for Animal Welfare, I sincerely hope to contribute to the complete abolition of cruelty to animals.

# Part One
# All about Aromatherapy

◆◇◆◇◆◇◆◇◆◇◆◇◆◇◆◇◆◇◆◇◆◇◆◇◆◇◆◇◆◇◆◇◆◇◆◇◆◇◆◇◆◇◆◇

# ◆ What Is Aromatherapy?

Aromatherapy is a subject with a great deal of appeal, but sadly it is surrounded by a lot of confusion and misunderstanding, leaving most people in a state of ignorance. This book may hopefully help the reader to be better informed.

Sometimes called 'Essential Oil Therapy', 'Osmotherapy' or 'Aromacology', aromatherapy is a truly holistic therapy, treating the body, mind and spirit by using essential oils extracted from plants.

The art of aromatherapy is rooted in the most ancient healing practices, dating back thousands of years when early peoples first discovered the medicinal properties or plants.

These days the widespread dissatisfaction with Western medicine and a leaning towards natural cures have caused many people to turn to complementary medicine such as aromatherapy for their physical, mental and emotional health.

Although the information in this book is based mainly on over 25 years of my own personal experience, a good deal of it is supported by the latest scientific findings that have grown out of considerable research into the medicinal properties of essential oils.

In aromatherapy treatments, essential oils are applied externally, but their penetrative power is so great that they act on the internal organs. Essential oils are like the blood running through our veins or the spirit of the plant; properly preserved, they have their own life-force and vibrational quality, which can be so healing when correctly used.

The subtle healing properties of essential oils are on a higher plane than chemical drugs, having a much more powerful effect on the psyche and the emotions. Essential oils offer a gentle and sensitive alternative to the dangers of synthetic drugs, which have caused an increasing number of adverse side-effects, allergic reactions, drug-dependence and addictions among patients.

The most important property of essential oils is the balancing effect they have on the body, since an imbalanced state in the body is the surest way of developing disease. Essential oils also have a very wide range of therapeutic properties, and there are a great many ailments that can be treated by these most natural of all plant medicines.

There are a wide variety of ways of using essential oils. The most important method of treatment is by diluting the essential oils in a vegetable 'carrier oil' and massaging the whole body, thus combining the beneficial effects of essential oils with the power of touch.

Another method of treatment is by adding the essential oils to a warm bath. This is a good supplement to massage treatments. The oils can also be used in burners for vaporization, inhalation, or as room fresheners. This method of treatment is particularly good for respiratory problems or when there is an infectious disease. For topical application, hot and cold compresses and creams are very useful ways of using the oils. In some cases, the essential oils can be applied neat. (More about all these methods in later chapters.)

Aromatherapy can be used to complement Western medicine or other forms of alternative therapy, as it often combines to great advantage with these other forms of treatment. It is truly the most wonderful and pleasant path to health and well-being.

# ◆ What Are Essential Oils?

Essential oils are quite different from vegetable oils. They are highly volatile and odorous, and therefore evaporate quickly when exposed to the air. Having a consistency more like water than oil, essential oils are different from vegetable oils in that they are not greasy and will not generally stain the way vegetable oils can. They are insoluble in water but soluble in alcohol, ether, and vegetable oils.

Most essential oils are clear or pale yellow, but a few are coloured, such as bergamot (green), chamomile (blue), patchouli (amber), bay (brown) and mandarin (golden). Chemically they are very complex, consisting of alcohols, esters, ketones, aldehydes and terpenes. Some oils contain more than 200 constituents.

These essential oils occur in all parts of the plants: the leaves, flowers, fruits, twigs, bark, wood, roots and resins. They occur in the plant tissues as tiny odiferous droplets in special secretory sacs at concentrations ranging from about 0.01 per cent to 10 per cent.

Although called 'essential oils', they are not in fact essential to plant life. The function of essential oils in plants is uncertain; some experts believe them to be waste products.

There are hundreds of aromatic plants, but only some are used for the extraction of essential oils on a commercial scale. The plants come from every conceivable part of the globe, and most are collected and distilled in their country of origin.

Plants, like all living things, are influenced by the conditions in which they grow. Aromatic plants are particularly sensitive to their growing conditions. The chemical composition of the oils produced in the plants, which determines their fragrance, is affected by factors such as the type of soil, altitude, temperature and humidity, as determined by the amount of sunshine and rainfall to which the plants are exposed.

In addition to these factors, the time of harvesting and the method of extraction also affect the final fragrance of the essential oils.

It is important to collect the plants for extraction at specific times to get the most oil of the best quality. Depending on the weather, time of year or even in which year they were gathered, different batches of the same essential oil may smell slightly different from each other. As well as the fragrance, the colour of the oils may also vary slightly.

Very often in the essential oil industry, which supplies mainly the perfume industry, when changes in the fragrance of the essential oils occur, they are adjusted by adding synthetic compounds to the natural oils to make them meet the industry standard.

In aromatherapy, the addition of synthetic chemicals to a natural essential oil is unacceptable; it compromises the oil's therapeutic properties. Therefore, when selecting essential oils for aromatherapy, all oils adulterated with synthetic chemicals are excluded even though they may smell more desirable to those who are unaware of the adulteration.

For this reason, there may be occasions when the natural essential oils differ perceptibly from their usual fragrance. The difference in smell is a small, tolerable compromise to ensure that the more important therapeutic properties are preserved.

Essential oils are used in three classes of consumer goods:

1. foods – as natural flavourings (e.g. rosemary, sage, lemon, parsley, fennel and caraway)
2. toiletries – in cosmetics and perfumes (e.g. peppermint, chamomile, neroli and rose)
3. medicines – as therapeutic agents (e.g. clove, eucalyptus, camphor and benzoin).

# ◆ Vegetable Oils

Vegetable oils (sometimes called fixed oils) act as carriers for essential oils for body, face and hair care. They have a greasy texture, making them easy to apply for massage. As with essential oils, keep your bottles of vegetable oil in a cool, dark place with the lids tightly secured. Although vegetable oils are not volatile, they can oxidize and turn rancid if they are not kept in the correct conditions. For personal use it is best to purchase them in small quantities of about 50 – 100 ml.

Vegetable oils have good skin penetration, leaving the skin nourished and feeling soft and supple. It is important that only pure, cold-pressed oils are used. After the initial cold-pressing, extractions are obtained by heat or solvent processing, which produces oils of inferior quality.

Mineral oil (baby oil) is not recommended because it is not absorbed by the skin but remains on the surface.

There are a variety of vegetable oils that can be purchased. However, below I have listed the oils which are most popular in aromatherapy.

## Almond Oil, Sweet (Prunus amygdalus)
Almond trees are found in the Mediterranean region. The oil is extracted from the kernel. It contains vitamin D and is good in treating dry and brittle nails. Almond is a popular oil and one of the least expensive used in massage. For a richer blend, it mixes well with avocado or jojoba.

## *Avocado Oil* (Persea americana)

Avocado trees are found in America and the Mediterranean countries. The oil is extracted from the flesh of the avocado. It is rich in vitamins A and D. Avocado is a nourishing oil with a good, rich texture. It is excellent for dry and dehydrated skins and has a good absorption rate.

Sometimes a good quality avocado oil may appear to be cloudy. This is not an indication of inferior quality, quite the reverse. In the winter months, the oil can start to solidify. By placing your oil in a warm room or holding the bottle between your hands, the oil will soon return to normal and become liquid again.

## *Evening Primrose Oil* (Oenothera biennis)

The evening primrose plant from North America is now widely grown all over Europe. The oil is extracted from the seeds. It has a high content of polyunsaturates and contains a large proportion of linoleic acid; it is also rich in gamma-linolenic acid (average 7.10 per cent). Evening primrose improves many skin problems such as rashes, dry skin, eczema and psoriasis. Use this oil on its own or, if preferred, blend with another oil such as jojoba. Once the bottle is opened, evening primrose has a very short life (up to two months). The oil can be purchased in 10-ml bottles.

## *Grapeseed Oil* (Vitis vinifera)

The grapevine is widely grown in the wine-producing regions of Europe. Grapeseed oil is extracted from the grape pips. This oil has a light texture and is a very popular oil used in massage. Like almond, it is one of the least expensive oils. Mixing it with either almond, avocado or peach kernel oils makes it a more suitable blend for use in aromatherapy massage.

## *Jojoba Oil* (Simmondsia chinensis)

The jojoba (pronounced ho-ho-ba) bush is an evergreen found in North America. The oil is extracted from the bean. It is rich in vitamin E and is a unique liquid wax used as an oil. It is fine, penetrating, stable and long-lasting. Jojoba can be used as a face moisturizer or as a more luxurious oil for massage. Jojoba has a very close chemical composition to the skin's own sebum. It is suitable for all skin types, beneficial for spotty and acne conditions, and is good for sensitive and oily skin. As it combines well with the sebum, it also helps to unclog the pores and remove any embedded grime. Jojoba works to condition and restore the health of the hair. Because of its fine texture, it is easy to wash out and is ideal for combating dandruff and dry scalp.

Widely used in the cosmetic industry for face and bath preparations, jojoba is an emollient for helping with eczema and psoriasis. Similar to avocado, jojoba turns completely solid in cold temperatures but will become liquid again when warmed.

## *Peach Kernel* (Prunus persica)

The peach tree is widely grown in Europe and North America. The oil is extracted from the kernel and contains essential fatty acids and vitamins A and E. It is an excellent oil for the face, encouraging suppleness and elasticity. It can be added to grapeseed or almond to enrich your massage blend.

## *Wheatgerm Oil* (Triticum vulgare)

Wheatgerm oil is extracted from the germ of the wheat kernel. It is very rich in texture and high in vitamin E; it is useful in reducing scar tissue and stretch marks. It is not suitable for use on its own for massage due to its thick texture and strong wheat odour. However, it is a natural anti-oxidant; adding 2–5 per cent of wheatgerm to your blends will preserve them for long periods of time.

# ◆ What Aromatherapy Can Do for You

Aromatherapy treatments using essential oils provide us with a whole range of benefits. They can help with many common disorders in a holistic way. Together with a healthy lifestyle, aromatherapy can get to the root of an illness even before symptoms develop.

Essential oils, like other plant remedies, have a long tradition of providing a variety of therapeutic benefits. Many of these benefits known of traditionally have recently been confirmed by modern scientific research.

Aromatherapy treatments have psycho-therapeutic benefits as well as affecting the physical state of the body. When the essential oils are used, either through massage, in a bath or by inhalation, the aroma will influence your psyche while the oils work on the tissues and organs of your body.

Essential oils are readily absorbed through the skin and carried to all parts of the body. Before they are finally eliminated by the body, the oils will continue to influence your system for several hours to several days (the length of time differs from person to person).

The oils are absorbed through the skin via the hair follicles which contain the oily substance, sebum. The sebum has a strong affinity with the essential oils and the oils are allowed to diffuse into the blood and the lymph. This process usually takes between one and six hours. (It is advisable not to shower during this time).

Particularly when used in treatment by massage, the aroma of the essential oils is combined with direct physical contact and produces the combined therapeutic benefits of both the sense of smell and touch. This unique combination causes powerful responses throughout the whole person, physically and emotionally.

Physiologically, the essential oils have an influence on the functions of the organs and tissues as well as on the nervous systems controlling the organs and tissues. They also have hormone-like actions and can help to regulate the endocrine system. Additionally, the oils have both antiseptic and antimicrobial actions, as well as the ability to stimulate the immune system to function more actively.

Although some essential oils have quite specific effects on the body, most of the oils have a very wide range of properties that overlap with each other. It is only with long experience of working closely with the oils that it is possible to choose the best essential oils for a particular condition.

The aroma of the oils directly affects our moods and emotions, and sometimes our short and long-term memory. Together with a wide range of physiological benefits, the aroma can help with emotional upsets such as depression, anxiety, nervous tension, anger, apathy, confusion, indecision, fear, grief, hypersensitivity, impatience, irritability, panic and hysteria. Treatments with essential oils are therefore very helpful for all sorts of stress-related problems, so common in our modern life.

Aromatherapy can benefit everyone, from babies to children, men, women and the elderly; helping in sickness and preventing disease. Regular treatments with essential oils will contribute to a dramatic improvement in general health and well-being, increasing vitality and giving you healthy-looking skin. Quite simply, aromatherapy works by influencing the body, mind and spirit all at the same time. When practised in a holistic way, aromatherapy treatments bring together the complete healing process.

# ♦ A Brief History of Aromatherapy

Aromatherapy has a very long history. As early as 3000 to 2000 BC (the golden age of ancient Egypt during the 12th dynasty) cosmetics were highly developed, involving the use of kohl as mascara for the eyes, various ointments and unguents to beautify the skin, and henna to colour the hair and nails. Many of the preparations during this period contained fragrances – the contents of ornate pots and jars, mostly made of alabaster or stone, can still be seen preserved in modern museums.

The spectacular tomb of Tutankhamen, built in 1350 BC, contained such vases and jars of scented unguents. The tomb was opened by archaeologists in 1922 to an astounded world audience. There are also papyri recording the medicinal properties of herbs dating back to the reign of Khufu, around 2800 BC. The Ebers papyrus includes many recipes for different treatments.

One of the famed perfumes of the Egyptians, Kyphi, is said to have contained the following aromatics: calamus, cassia, cinnamon, citronella, juniper, myrrh and peppermint. Besides the Egyptians, the Babylonians also used aromatics widely. Cedarwood is mentioned as one of the prized aromatics, recorded on clay tablets dating back to 1800 BC.

When Julius Caesar and Mark Anthony fell in love with the famous Egyptian queen, Cleopatra, her lavish use of aromatics was credited with the seduction of both men.

The Chinese were another people at the very height of civilization. The oldest medical text, written by Huang Ti and called *The Yellow Emperor's Classic of Internal Medicine*, deals with the causes

12

and treatment of diseases and includes several medicinal herbs.

The Hebrew Old Testament makes several references to aromatics. Moses was given a recipe for making a holy anointing oil consisting of myrrh, cinnamon, cassia and calamus. Solomon wrote much beautiful poetry which contained descriptions of aromatic herbs such as myrrh, lily, rose, spikenard, saffron, calamus, cinnamon, frankincense and aloe.

The use of aromatic medicines and cosmetics was as prevalent in Greece as in Egypt. The Greek physician Hippocrates from the island of Kos, who lived from 460 to 377 BC, is regarded as the father of modern medicine. He also started a medical school that became famous during his own time. Among his writings, several aromatic herbs are mentioned, including aniseed, caraway, coriander, cumin, fennel and thyme. Even today, many people including medical practitioners from all over the world visit the famous island of Kos as a place of historical interest.

Another Greek writer, Theophrastus, recognized the medicinal properties of perfumes and included many aromatic plants in his botanical writings. Other writers such as Herodotus and Democretus elaborated on the art of perfumery.

In the New Testament, the old Greek writers mention the account of Mary Magdalene pouring fragrant ointment of spikenard on Jesus' feet and wiping them with her hair. Roy Genders, a modern-day writer on perfumery, tells us that among the most famous Greek perfumes was Megaleion, a mixture of myrrh, cinnamon and cassia added to balanos oil.

The Romans were even more lavish in their use of aromatics than the Greeks. Renowned for their scented baths, the Romans also used perfume to massage their bodies and scent their hair. These aromatics were enclosed in bottles of alabaster and kept in ivory boxes.

The writings of Galen were so influential that they dominated herbal medicine in Europe until the Middle Ages, his formulas being called 'galenic'. Galen described many preparations involving aromatics, including the cold cream still used in modern cosmetics.

Trading between the Far East and Europe was carried out mainly by the Arabs, and among the commodities were the exotic aromatics from India and China such as jasmine, sandalwood, cinnamon, cassia and camphor. The Arabs are also credited with the discovery of distillation. Among the Arabs, one of the most outstanding physicians was Avicenna, who wrote several standard works on medicine. His accounts cover over 800 medicinal plants and include aromatic herbs such as rose, lavender and chamomile.

The history of aromatics in India is equally ancient, with sandalwood, rose, jasmine and spikenard recorded in early Ayurvedic writings.

In Europe, aromatic herbs were widely used during the great plague of the Middle Ages. Public fires fuelled with pine wood, and personal fumigation using incense of various gums and resins offered protection from the contagion due to their strong antiseptic properties.

The golden age of English herbalism, in the seventeenth century, saw the production of many herbals and books about aromatics – some of which are still influential today. Two of the most popular herbals of this period are from John Gerard and Nicholas Culpepper. Others were written by Turner, Parkinson and Miller. Culpepper translated the official Latin herbal texts of his time into English for the common people, and also included information on astrology, linking each herb with a 'ruling planet'.

In the eighteenth century Johann Maria Farina formulated the toilet water, Eau de Cologne (originally called 'Kolnisches Wasser'), to this day well known for its cooling, refreshing, deodorant and antiseptic properties. Eau de Cologne is made from several citrus essential oils including bergamot and neroli, as well as lavender and rosemary.

Another famous aromatic water is Hungary Water, named after Queen Elizabeth of Hungary. This preparation is quite similar to Eau de Cologne in composition but also includes rose water and is based very much on rosemary essential oil.

In 1928 the first book on aromatherapy was published by René Maurice Gattefossé, a French chemist who worked with essential oils. In 1964 another Frenchman, Dr Jean Valnet, who used essential oils in the treatment of his patients, wrote a book on aromatherapy.

Marguérite Maury, an Austrian biochemist, pioneered using essential oils in massage. She made a thorough study of the way aromatics worked both physically and emotionally. Her work has been of great value. In 1962, Mme Maury was awarded the 'Prix International d'Esthetique et Cosmetologie' in recognition of her contributions to this field.

And now to the present time ...

# ◆ Extraction Methods

In ancient times, aromatics were obtained in two ways:

1.  maceration – soaking the plant materials in a vegetable base oil
2.  enfleurage – placing flower petals on purified animal fats.

However, it was only possible to obtain pure essential oils with the discovery of distillation, first mentioned in Europe by a Spaniard called Arnold de Vilanova in around the thirteenth century, although the Arabs have since been credited with its discovery much earlier.

These days there are several possible methods of extracting pure essential oils. Three of the most important methods are steam distillation, expression, and solvent extraction.

## Steam Distillation

The most important and widely used method of extraction is steam distillation. This method involves placing the plant material on a grid inside a distillation vat and passing steam under pressure from beneath the vessel.

The heat of the steam causes the cell walls of the leaves, twigs, berries and other parts of the plant in which the essential oil is stored to break down and release the essential oil as a vapour. To obtain the maximum yield some plants are distilled immediately after harvesting, while those which benefit from being left to dry are distilled after several days' time.

This essential oil vapour is passed together with the steam through cooling tanks which cause the vapour to condense so that it can be collected. When both the steam and essential oil vapour are cooled, the essential oil usually floats on the water in the collecting tanks, as most essential oils are lighter than water. The essential oils are then separated out.

The essential oil can impart some of its fragrance to the distillation water; this water can be sold off separately as floral or herbal water, sometimes also called hydrolate.

Steam distillation is still the most economical method of extraction. The distillation stills in modern distilleries are made of stainless steel to avoid contamination and produce better quality oils.

## Expression

This form of extraction applies only to citrus oils. The peel of all citrus fruits is full of oil glands containing globules of essential oils. The peel is separated from the pulp, which contains the juice. This peel is then squeezed by simple pressure to press out the essential oil. Some juice will be extracted from the pith together with the oil. The solution is left to stand so that the oil and juice separate; the oil is then collected. The expression method was formerly performed by hand but is now done by machine on a much larger scale.

## Solvent Extraction

The final products of solvent extraction are called absolutes, concretes and resinoids. This method of extraction is used mainly for some of the finest flowers.

The flower petals are placed in a sealed container. Liquid solvent is then allowed to flow over the flowers and completely cover them. The solvent will slowly dissolve the essential oils from the petals. This solution is collected and the solvent is then distilled off and returned to its tank to be re-used. The solvents normally used are petroleum ether or hexane.

On separation, a semi-solid aromatic material called a concrete is left. The concrete contains some of the natural waxes found in the plant. To remove the waxes and other non-aromatic materials, the concrete is shaken with alcohol; when the alcohol is distilled off, a coloured liquid is left – this is called an absolute.

Resinoids are similar to concretes but are extracted from the resins that exude from trees rather than from the flowers.

# ◆ Buying, Storing and Caring for Essential Oils

## Buying Essential Oils

When buying your essential oils it is preferable to be in contact with a supplier specializing in aromatherapy, concerned with the importance of purity and available for queries. Many brands are now flooding the country, some of which are adulterated. Only pure essential oils will give the desired therapeutic effects; synthetics cannot achieve these results.

Occasionally, essential oils can be found labelled as organic. The term 'organic' implies that the plant in cultivation is grown without the use of fertilizers and insecticides. There are a few essential oils that are organically produced, but it would be inaccurate to say that all or most are. It would be impossible to inspect growing methods comprehensively, as the plants are grown in various regions all over the world.

Essential oils are volatile, so it is important to avoid bottles which can be opened by shoppers, and to protect against contamination. It would help to buy from shops that have a range of testers.

Generally it is best not to evaluate more than about six oils at any one time, as the nose soon gets 'saturated' from exposure to too many different odours. When testing, choose an area free from odours; clear your nose before and between testing each oil. Be careful not to inhale too deeply, as some of the oils can be quite overpowering. Care should be taken that your skin does not come into contact with the undiluted oils.

Essential oils should always be supplied in dark bottles, with either an inserted dropper or a separate glass rod dropper with a rubber teat called a pipette. A 10-ml bottle of essential oil will contain approximately 200 drops. The more expensive essential oils, such as rose, neroli, jasmine, melissa, and Roman and German chamomiles, can be purchased in 5-ml or 2½-ml sizes.

## Storing Essential Oils

Essential oils are delicate substances and are affected by strong light, heat, air and moisture. For protection they are best kept in a cool, dry and dark place. The bathroom is not suitable as it is a place of high humidity. Avoid storing near heat such as radiators or cookers. Ideally, a cupboard in the bedroom would be suitable.

## Caring for Essential Oils

Do not transfer your essential oils to plastic bottles, as the plastic will interact with the chemical makeup of the essential oils and the oils will cause the plastic to deteriorate. Wooden chests to carry 10 to 24 bottles can be purchased; they are ideal for storing and carrying essential oils.

# ✦ Handling and Mixing Essential Oils

## Handling Essential Oils

Using bottles with in-built glass pipettes has many advantages when handling essential oils. You will have more control than with an inserted dropper and be able to dispense an accurate amount of essential oil. A pipette also makes it easier to remove the last few drops from the bottom of a bottle.

Empty glass bottles are available in various sizes. A 30-ml bottle is a good size for body massage, a 10-ml bottle for face massage. A small funnel can be useful for transferring your vegetable oils to smaller bottles. These can be obtained at your health shop or chemist. Be especially careful to replace the right pipette into the correct bottle, otherwise you will contaminate your oils with different odours. Also remember to check that you have screwed the correct tops securely on each bottle after use.

The various essential oils have different viscosities: some (such as peppermint and rosemary) are very light, almost like water, while others (such as patchouli and myrrh) are thick like syrup. Be especially careful with the lighter, watery essential oils, as some may pour out of the inserted dropper very quickly, while some of the heavier oils may take a longer time to come out and can eventually clog up the hole. The citrus oils have a shorter life than some of the other essential oils. Once opened (especially lemon, grapefruit or orange), they can turn cloudy as they start to deteriorate. If using a glass pipette, you will be able to notice this change. This also applies to any changes in either the colour or texture of all the essential oils; it is almost impossible to see these changes through the amber glass of the bottles they come in.

If you are using bottles with a separate pipette, make sure that they are always kept in an upright position so that the oil will not get into contact with the rubber teat, as some essential oils react with rubber. It is also advisable to squeeze out all the oil from the pipette before replacing it in the bottle.

## Mixing Essential Oils

Mixing essential oils is not complicated but there are a few basic rules to follow. Always use clean, dry, glass bottles and measuring equipment, and mix your oils on a worktop that is easily washable. Essential oils can damage varnished or plastic surfaces – have paper tissues or a towel handy to mop up any spillages.

Before you start mixing your essential oils, first decide how much base oil you will need. Fill your bottle with the required amount of vegetable oil. Choose no more than three essential oils and first write down the names of the essential oils you are going to use and the required number of drops of each essential oil you are using.

When blending essential oils, the dilution used can vary from 1 per cent to 5 per cent depending on the person and condition being treated. The usual strength is 2 per cent, which means mixing 1 drop of essential oil to every 2 ml of vegetable oil. If using a 10-ml bottle of vegetable oil, the total amount of essential oil is 5 drops. If using a 50-ml bottle of vegetable oil, add a total of 25 drops of essential oil. This applies whether you are using just one essential oil or a combination of two or three different essential oils.

If you are using a 30-ml bottle for a body massage, add 25 ml of your chosen vegetable oil to the empty bottle. Do not fill the oil to the top of the bottle, to avoid any overflow and to leave a little room for your essential oils. The next step is to add your essential oils. For a therapeutic blend, about 12–15 drops are usually required. However, for a relaxing or refreshing and invigorating blend, a total of approximately 8 drops is sufficient.

Add to your bottle of base oil your first essential oil, making note of the number of drops used. Then add your second essential oil, again writing down the number of drops. Adding your third essential oil should balance the blend.

Shake the bottle so that the oils are blended well together. Remove the lid and smell the mix. Then rub a little of the mix on the back of your hand and smell it again.

Like perfume, it will smell differently on your skin. You may wish to correct your blend to keep one essential oil from dominating the others. For example, if you have added too much geranium or ylang-ylang, making the smell too sweet, you can rectify the blend by softening it with a few drops of sandalwood. If your blend smells too medicinal, again you can rectify the blend, this time by adding a few drops of orange; this will make the blend more acceptable to the nose and will save you having to waste your blends unnecessarily.

When you have made your blend, gently shake the bottle to ensure the oils are thoroughly mixed. Mix only the amount you require at any one time. If you wish to mix more than the required amount for future use, add approximately 2–5 per cent of wheatgerm to preserve your mix from turning rancid, unless you are using jojoba as a base.

When blending an oil for the face, or for young children, the amount of essential oil added to your vegetable oil should be halved, making it a 1 per cent dilution.

Mixing essential oils and creating your very own special formulas can be very exciting. However, it can also be very frustrating, especially when you are inexperienced and the final blend turns out not to be pleasing to your nose. Until you become more proficient with your own blending skills, I have provided a comprehensive range of recipes for all the common problems you may encounter in everyday life, and also for improving your general well-being (see Part 3).

# ♦ How Safe Are Essential Oils?

How often should you use essential oils? Obviously it is not recommended to use an inhalation each day of every week. You would only require an inhalation to treat a specific condition, and it would be sufficient to have two inhalations a day for up to four days at a time or when required.

Using a few drops of essential oils in the bath each day would have no adverse effects. The same applies to room vaporization. Blending essential oils into a base oil or cream to be used as a perfume would also have no adverse effects.

For a massage or direct application to the body, twice weekly should suffice. Applying essential oils to a specific part of the body to treat a problem may be carried out daily, until the condition clears. If the problem persists, consult your doctor.

In all the years that I have been involved in aromatherapy I can justifiably say that the only adverse reactions have been experienced by those few individuals who have had an allergic reaction or have used the essential oils in an improper manner.

All the oils that I have included in this book are easily available commercially and can be obtained from most health food shops. They are also safe if used properly by following my instructions in this book carefully.

During the last few years I have been very concerned by articles printed in the tabloid papers and magazines on how dangerous using essential oils can be. These articles tended to be horror stories without any research basis. Finally, in 1993 my company, Natural by Nature Oils, financed and published 'A Safety Guide on the Use of Essential Oils' to address this adverse publicity.

Essential oils are very concentrated and should be used with care!

**Precautions:**

- Do not use undiluted essential oils on the skin (except where indicated).
- Keep out of the reach of children.
- Keep away from the eyes. If essential oils have accidentally touched the eyes, splash the eyes immediately with tepid water. If a burning sensation occurs, seek medical advice. Do not drop vegetable oils into the eyes to try to remedy the situation, as they are greasy and will worsen the problem.
- Some people may have an allergic reaction to essential oils.
- Extra precautions should be taken during pregnancy regarding the use of essential oils (especially during the first few months).
- Do not take essential oils internally.
- Do not apply essential oils when sunbathing.
- Certain essential oils (such as camphor, eucalyptus and peppermint) should not be used while taking homoeopathic medicines, as these oils counteract the effects of homoeopathic remedies.
- When using essential oils in the bath, swirl the water well to help disperse the oils. For babies and young children, or if you have sensitive skin, it is best to disperse your essential oils in a teaspoonful of jojoba oil first. Using essential oils in the bath without blending them with a base oil first can in time discolour fibreglass baths.

# ◆ An Introduction to Massage

Massage is as old as the human race, and must be the oldest form of complementary medicine. To touch is to care; through massage we become aware of our ability to heal and help many stress-related problems.

Manuscripts have been found from the ancient civilizations of China, Egypt and India referring to massage to cure and heal. There are many references to massage written by the ancient Romans and Greeks. The earliest book to mention massage dates back to 2700 BC. Hippocrates used massage on his patients, emphasizing the importance of pressure and technique to obtain the desired effect.

Here I give you just a short introduction to massage. Although I would have liked to write on this further, a whole book is needed on the subject – and indeed there are some excellent books already available; I have listed a few which I am sure you will enjoy at the back of this book.

## Getting Prepared

The comfort of your partner is of utmost importance, as you need to ensure complete relaxation. To create the right conditions, you need to start by collecting the basic tools, getting the required atmosphere and getting your room prepared.

Preheat the room ensuring that the temperature is warm enough – your partner will be undressed and body temperature drops quickly while lying still. Parts of the body you will be massaging will be exposed for a period of time. Warm towels should be available to cover the areas you are not working on.

Privacy is important: Take the telephone off the hook and, if you have pets, put them in another room or you may find them joining in!

Background music is also important: Choose something that you both enjoy, but make sure the music has flowing rhythms and is right for that relaxing mood. Dim the lights or light candles. Do not forget to use your essential oil burner. The room should be well ventilated and free from any unwanted odours of cooking or smoke.

Wear appropriate clothing. Do not wear long baggy sleeves, as they will get in the way. Wear something light as you will also get hot. Your partner may be completely undressed or may, for modesty's sake, prefer to keep her underwear on. To avoid getting your partner's hair oily it should be tied back away from her face and neck. You should also tie back your own hair to prevent it getting in the way when you bend over to do the massage. Jewellery can get in the way and may scratch, so it is best removed. Check that your fingernails are not too long.

The easiest way to do a massage is on a massage table. However, there is no need to be disappointed if you do not own one. You can achieve a wonderful massage working on the floor (a bed is not firm enough to make a suitable substitute). You will need a temporary working surface. A large piece of foam rubber padding will be sufficient. Do ensure that the padding is wide enough as you will be kneeling and sitting alongside your partner. Alternatively, make a suitable surface with blankets or sleeping bags. Cover this makeshift massage table with towels; use additional folded towels to give support to the lower back and behind the knees and calves. A folded towel will also give a slight lift to the back of the head.

There are some points to consider before mixing, to help you mix the correct amount of oil. You may have a partner who is hairy, of above-average size or who has dry skin. You may find while practising that you will be using more oil than is usually required. Be careful and try not to turn your partner into a sardine! However, too little oil can have the opposite effect by dragging the skin. At first your massage movements will be a little clumsy and your hands will be sliding all over the place. But do not worry; with practice your movements will become more co-ordinated.

Remember to keep your hands in contact with your partner's body at all times.

## Giving a Massage

Before you start, your hands should be warm and the oil at room temperature.

You are now ready to start your massage, and I will try and help to guide you through some basic massage techniques. Try keeping a good posture. This can be difficult working on the floor, so every now and then you may need to have a stretch.

Start by kneeling to the upper left side of your partner. Place your hands gently onto the centre of her back. This will engage your contact.

Pour a little of your prepared oil into the cupped palm of your hand, then gently apply the oil evenly over the surface of your partner's back and shoulders. Remember to try and mould your hands to the contours of her body.

Now place both hands at the base of your partner's lower back, in the centre, with your fingers pointing towards her head. Make a sweeping motion up to her neck, keeping your palms flat. Then, parting your hands, move them up in opposite directions out and over her shoulders.

Bring your hands back down to the base of your partner's back and repeat the movement 4–5 times. This movement is called *effleurage*; use it before and after finishing each section of the body.

Your next movement can start on the far side of the lower back with your right hand flat, reinforced by your left hand on top. Move in firm clockwise circles up the side to the top of the shoulder, then move across to repeat the movement going down on the near side in an anti-clockwise direction.

Keep your body relaxed and your movements flowing.

**Thumb kneading:** Again, begin at the base of the spine and with firm, even pressure, using the pads of your thumbs, make slow circular movements moving outwards, simultaneously on each side of the spine.

For the next movement you will only be using one hand. Place the hand you are not using on your partner's left shoulder, and glide your other hand to the nape of her neck, just below the hairline. With your thumb and fingers, very gently squeeze and lift the muscle in an upward movement. Do this about six times. Next, with your fingers and thumbs using small circular movements, work around the shoulder blades, releasing tension and all those tight knots that have accumulated over a period of time.

When you have finished, keep your partner well covered with towels and allow a few minutes for her to savour the delights of your wonderful massage!

You may now let your pets in, as by now they will be feeling very envious!

## General Benefits of Massage

- stimulates circulation
- stimulates the immune system
- eases tense muscles and muscular pain
- enhances mental and physical relaxation
- increases muscle flexibility and adds tone to slack muscles
- breaks down fat deposits and waste products in the tissues
- promotes relaxation and restful sleep
- promotes a feeling of well-being and comfort
- creates a feeling of being cared for
- helps to remove inhibitions.

## General Precautions in Massage

*Do not massage:*

- any painful areas
- swollen and inflamed joints
- eruptions and skin inflammation
- areas of eczema or psoriasis
- areas of thrombosis and phlebitis
- recent fractures and broken bones
- contagious or infectious skin conditions
- unrecognized tumours (lumps and bumps)
- recent scar tissue
- directly on varicose veins (massaging around the veins, however, will help to drain the blood from the varicose areas)
- if your partner has a fever
- if your partner is suffering from a migraine (massage can over-stimulate the head)
- if she is in the first 2–3 days of menstruation (as massage may increase the blood flow).

- Be especially careful during the first few months of pregnancy.
- Be gentle with the elderly, young children and babies.
- In cases of cancer, cardio-vascular conditions such as high-blood pressure, angina pectoris or any other serious conditions, always consult your doctor first.

A good 'rule of thumb' is:
   WHEN IN DOUBT – DON'T!

# ◆ Treatments with Water and Essential Oils

## Baths

A most pleasurable way of using essential oils is in your daily bath, as this has a therapeutic effect on both mind and body. Choose one or a combination of two or three essential oils, using a total of up to 8 drops of essential oil.

A morning soak will revitalize and refresh you for that hectic day ahead, use the refreshing and stimulating essential oils such as rosemary and bergamot. Bathing before bedtime will help to give a restful night's sleep provided you use the relaxing and sedative essential oils such as lavender and frankincense. Baths are also beneficial for treating muscular pain and tension.

After running your bath water and ensuring that the water is not too hot (as this will only make the vapours from the oil evaporate quickly), before getting in swirl the water so the oils are evenly dispersed. Relax and soak for 10 to 15 minutes, all the while inhaling the aroma of the essential oils.

Dry skin, eczema and psoriasis can be aggravated by water and it is advisable to add a little jojoba oil to your bath water. This same method can be used for sensitive skin and for children and babies. Stir your blend of jojoba and essential oils before adding it to the bath water. For sensitive skin and for children's baths, use only 2 or 3 drops of essential oils.

The following list of essential oils may irritate the skin. Use in a lower concentration and blend with a little jojoba oil first:

| anise | clove | nutmeg |
|---|---|---|
| basil | cumin | peppermint |
| camphor | hyssop | sage |
| cinnamon | lemongrass | thyme |
| citronella | melissa | the citrus essential oils. |

It is best for the thicker essential oils (such as benzoin, myrrh, sandalwood and vetivert) to be blended with a little jojoba oil, as this will help to stop them from sinking to the bottom of the bath or sticking to the surface of the bathtub.

# Footbaths

When a bath is not available or convenient, footbaths can be very helpful. Add up to 6 drops of essential oil to a bowl of warm water and soak the feet for approximately 10 minutes. Essential oils penetrate through the feet very quickly and are good for conditions such as colds, varicose veins, Athlete's foot, sore and painful feet, and swollen ankles.

# Hot and Cold Compresses

Compresses are an effective way of alleviating many conditions. For a large area, add approximately 5–8 drops of essential oil to a basin filled with hot or cold water; for a smaller area, add 2–4 drops of essential oil to a small bowl or dish of water. Agitate the water to help disperse the essential oils evenly. Place a cotton flannel or handkerchief on top of the water, which will collect the floating oil. Gently squeeze out any excess water and apply to the affected area. Wrap a towel or bandage over the compress and leave until the compress reaches body temperature, then repeat the process. A hot compress is effective for rheumatic, menstrual, back or abdominal pains. Urinary problems such as cystitis can be helped by this method. Abscess, earache and toothache can also benefit. Use a cold compress for sunburn, headache, varicose veins and bruises. It will also help to reduce inflammation caused by sprains and to alleviate the pain of hot and swollen areas.

## Sauna and Steam Rooms

You will always get a wonderful and clean feeling after having a sauna or steam in combination with essential oils. The winter months are a time for colds and blocked noses, respiratory and bronchial troubles. Using a mixture of essential oils such as pine, eucalyptus, camphor and cajeput is a good antiviral mix. Do not add essential oils directly onto the stones. Always make sure they are thoroughly mixed with the water in your bucket, stirring it with a ladle before splashing it onto the stones.

For the steam room it is not advisable to put essential oils into your tank, as most are made of plastic and in time the oils may damage an expensive part of the system. It is better to place a bowl of water containing the essential oils in the corner of the steam room.

## Vaporization and Room Fresheners

Essential oil burners, sometimes called vaporizers, are available in all sorts of shapes and sizes. You simply add water and approximately 12–15 drops of your chosen oils, depending on the size of the room (additional oils can be added as required).

Choose a burner that can hold a lot of water – the more water it holds, the longer its vaporizing action will last. (Never let the water run dry, as your burner might crack). The candle inserted in or placed under the burner gently warms the water and oil, which evaporates, creating the desired atmosphere. Depending on the essential oils used, this can be stimulating and head-clearing, or calming and relaxing. Burners are very beneficial to asthma and hayfever sufferers, and purify the air to help prevent the spread of infection. They also make ideal room fresheners and are handy for getting rid of unpleasant odours.

Additionally, they make good insect repellents.

If you cannot keep a watchful eye on your burner, another alternative is an electric vaporizer, for which no candle is needed. These are more expensive but are a safer method, especially for use in a child's room.

# Steam Inhalation

Inhalation is a method of introducing essential oils to the lungs via the nose and throat. This can be beneficial for respiratory problems, sinus congestion, colds, flu, coughs, catarrh and sore throats. This method can be used once or twice daily.

Add approximately 6 drops of either one or a combination of two or three oils to a bowl of near-boiling water, lean over the bowl and cover your head with a towel to prevent the vapours from escaping. This is also very effective for cleansing the pores of the face. Alternatively, an electric facial sauna can be used which will keep the water at a constant temperature. This method uses less water, so you need add only half the amount of essential oils needed for a steam inhalation.

The vapours from the oils can be very strong – keep your eyes closed. Inhale slowly at first, then gradually breathe deeper. Breathing through the mouth will benefit throat problems. The length of time necessary can vary from 2 minutes (if your skin is sensitive) up to 5 to 10 minutes maximum. It is not advisable to use steam treatments if you have broken veins, sunburn, psoriasis or eczema. Nor is it advisable to use steam inhalation during an asthma attack.

Inhalation can also be used by adding a few drops of essential oils to a handkerchief and sniffing at it regularly throughout the day. This is an effective way to relieve travel sickness and nausea. The same method can be used for keeping alert when travelling on long journeys, or the handkerchief can be placed by your pillow to help you get to sleep.

# Mouthwash and Gargle

This method is useful for sore throats, infected gums, mouth ulcers, fungal conditions and bad breath. It is also good for loss of voice. Half-fill a tumbler with boiled, cooled water, adding 2–3 drops of essential oil. Stir well before each mouthful. Do not swallow.

# Creams and Lotions

In addition to using vegetable oils as a base for essential oils, you can use a cream or lotion. Use a fragrance- and lanolin-free cream made from plant products. A lotion is best used if you need to apply essential oils over a large area. To stop the lotion from dragging the skin, add a small amount of jojoba or avocado oil. This also makes for a more nourishing blend.

Creams are ideal for creating your own moisturizers or perfumes. Add a small amount of jojoba, peach or avocado oil to obtain the consistency required for your skin type. For a dry complexion, add avocado. For problematic skin, add evening primrose.

Essential oils added to creams can be used for various skin problems such as Athlete's foot, cold sores, insect bites, spots, minor cuts and grazes, rashes, sunburn, psoriasis and eczema. If the oils are to be used as an antiseptic or to combat conditions such as thrush, they are easier to use with a cream as your base.

# Neat Application

It is not advisable to apply neat essential oils onto the skin. However, there are some exceptions. Minor burns, insect bites, warts, verrucas, nail-bed and pierced ear infections can be treated successfully in this way. Ensure that you avoid making contact with the surrounding, healthy skin.

When applying essential oils onto the face, for example to a spot or cold sore, first soak the tip of a cotton bud with water then add 2 drops of essential oil. This also applies to toothache and mouth ulcers. For Athlete's foot, soak the feet in water and tea tree. Then apply neat tea tree to the feet, not forgetting to dab the essential oil between the toes.

## Taking Essential Oils Internally

In the practice of aromatherapy we do not recommend taking essential oils internally. Essential oils are very concentrated and can be 100–1,000 times stronger than the herb they are obtained from. It is important to realize that essential oils can be irritating to the mucous membranes, and that they are only sparingly soluble in water.

*N.B.* – If you want to take a herb internally the best way is to drink the herbal tea, not to ingest the essential oil derived from that herb.

# ♦ Pot-pourri and Essential Oils

Pot-pourri is a mixture of dried leaves, flowers, twigs, spices, roots and essential oils. An abundance of plant material can be collected all year round from gardens or woods.

To make your own pot-pourri, it is best to gather the ingredients on a dry day. Dry your plant material on a flat surface or in net bags hanging in a dark, warm and airy place.

The spring and summer months bring a vast variety of aromatic herbs: thyme, sage, peppermint, rosemary, chamomile, verbena, marjoram, lavender and melissa are among the more common herbs found growing in many gardens.

Autumn brings a colourful mixture of leaves, twigs, seeds, berries and cones. These make a good decoration for the festive season, especially when woody essential oils are added.

In the winter months, look out for eucalyptus, juniper berries, bay, rosemary and pine.

For the kitchen, use different coloured peels of fruits (they can be dried in a microwave oven). Add to these the citrus essential oils for a zesty, fruity aroma.

Rose petals, stocks, feverfew, marigolds and freesia are among the many hundreds of flowers which can be dried and used to make a colourful table decoration. Add the floral essential oils to your mix.

If you are short of plant material, your local health food shop or supermarket will have a selection of herbs, spices, seeds and bark to choose from. Put the dried ingredients into a bowl and separately blend your essential oils. As a fixative, there are several essential oils to choose from, including vetivert, cedarwood, sandalwood, benzoin, myrrh and patchouli.

Add your blend of oils to the dried pot-pourri, carefully mixing your ingredients together and taking care not to crush any delicate leaves or petals. Your mixture should now be coated with a fine film of essential oils.

Cover the mixture with a lid to seal it, then leave for 5–7 days. This gives the ingredients a chance to mature. Pot-pourri can be used in a variety of ways and makes a wonderful gift. Bowls and decorative dishes filled with pot-pourri make a delightful table decoration while simultaneously giving your rooms a fragrant aroma. Top up with essential oils when required.

For a restful night, fill pillows with lavender oil and dried flowers. To keep moths at bay, hang or place sachets filled with clove buds and clove oil in your cupboards and drawers. Car pomanders can be filled with rosemary and basil herbs and oil to enliven the traveller on a long journey.

Bath sachets are another way of using essential oils and pot-pourri. Wrap your prepared mix in muslin and tie the bundle with a piece of string. This method is ideal for a fragrant or therapeutic soak. From a selection of fabrics, design different shapes and sizes to put your pot-pourri mix in. They make wonderful gifts for all occasions.

# Part Two

# Using Essential Oils

◆◇◆◇◆◇◆◇◆◇◆◇◆◇◆◇◆◇◆◇◆◇◆◇◆◇◆◇◆◇◆◇◆◇◆◇◆◇◆◇◆◇◆◇◆◇◆◇

# ◆ The General Effects of Essential Oils on the Different Body Systems

## The Digestive System

Problems of digestion usually affect the stomach, liver and gall-bladder. Improper eating may strain the digestive system and result in indigestion, causing spasm, colic, flatulence and constipation. Besides the wide range of herbal preparations to take internally, the external application of essential oils is also beneficial. Treatment is by local compress over the abdominal area and back massage over the lower spine region, with the following examples of essential oils:

- chamomile, caraway, melissa, sage, peppermint, anise, fennel, coriander and cumin – antispasmodic for painful spasms
- angelica, basil, peppermint, fennel, cardamon and anise – carminative for flatulence and dyspepsia
- clove, cinnamon, nutmeg, ginger and black pepper – stomachic to counter stomach acidity
- rosemary, peppermint, lemon and lime – hepatic for liver congestion
- peppermint and caraway – cholagogic for stimulating the gall-bladder to secrete bile
- bergamot, peppermint, basil, anise, angelica, orange and ginger – aperitifs for promoting appetite and the secretion of saliva
- fennel, camphor, peppermint, black pepper, marjoram and rosemary – mild laxatives to promote bowel movement.

# The Urinary System

This system is prone to infection. Essential oils are very helpful in dealing with urinary problems as they promote the flow of urine and have an antiseptic effect on urinary tract infections. Treatment is by massage of the lumbo-sacral region, compresses and hip baths, with the following examples of essential oils:

- juniper, lemon, celery, rosemary, fennel and parsley – diuretic (encourages the flow of urine)
- sandalwood, bergamot, tea tree and benzoin – antiseptic (for urinary tract infections).

# The Circulatory System

The heart and circulation are essential to the proper functioning of all the organs and tissues of the body. Problems of this system include high and low blood pressure, circulatory complaints, and weakness in the muscular contraction of the heart. Essential oils can be easily absorbed through the skin and mucous membranes into the blood. Treatment is by compress over the heart area, back massage over the dorsal region, and by aromatic baths with the following examples of essential oils:

- lavender, geranium, marjoram, clary sage, lemon, and ylang-ylang – hypotensive to reduce high blood pressure
- rosemary, camphor, thyme and cumin – hypertensive to raise lowered blood pressure
- hyssop and angelica – tonic to regulate blood pressure
- benzoin, cinnamon, black pepper, marjoram, cardamon, ginger and nutmeg – rubefacient to warm and stimulate the circulation
- rose, melissa, orange and neroli – antispasmodic action on the heart
- cypress – to combat constriction of the veins.

# The Respiratory System

The whole respiratory system, including the nose, throat and lungs, is prone to infection. Essential oils have excellent antiseptic properties and make very effective treatments for respiratory problems. Treatment is by inhalation complemented with back massage over the dorsal region and local compresses on the chest with the following examples of essential oils:

- cinnamon, thyme, tea tree, eucalyptus, pine, camphor, clove, lemon, peppermint, niaouli and cajeput – general antiseptics
- eucalyptus, camphor, pine, thyme, rosemary, hyssop, lemon, myrrh, cajeput and benzoin – expectorants to clear the respiratory tract of mucous
- clary sage, anise, hyssop, cypress, frankincense, rosemary and basil – antispasmodics for coughs.

# The Endocrine System

The endocrine glands which together form the endocrine system are responsible for regulating growth, metabolism and reproduction, by the production of hormones. Essential oils may either stimulate the endocrine glands to produce hormones, or act as some of the hormones themselves, having a direct regulating effect on the body. Treatment is by massage with the following examples of essential oils:

- basil, geranium, rosemary, sage and pine – stimulate the adrenal glands
- peppermint and jasmine – stimulate the pituitary gland
- rose, chamomile and clary sage – stimulate the reproductive glands
- fennel, anise, sage and angelica – oestrogenic effect
- fennel, anise and lemongrass – promote milk secretion
- sage, peppermint and parsley – reduce milk secretion.

# The Reproductive System

The reproductive system can be affected by hormonal changes and also by infection. Aromatherapy treatments help with complaints such as menstrual problems, genital infections and sexual difficulties. Some essential oils have an affinity with the reproductive system as they have a regulating and strengthening effect, others have useful antimicrobial actions. A few essential oils are also aphrodisiac, thereby helping with frigidity or impotence. Treatment is by massage over the lower abdomen and by hip baths with the following examples of essential oils:

- bergamot, sandalwood, tea tree, chamomile, myrrh, benzoin, cinnamon and lavender – antimicrobial and antiseptic
- juniper, fennel, parsley, celery, carrot, caraway, angelica, cypress, myrrh and marjoram – emmenagogic
- jasmine, ylang-ylang, neroli, rose, sandalwood, patchouli, vetivert and clary sage – aphrodisiac
- anise, basil, peppermint, melissa, marjoram, chamomile, lavender and rosemary – antispasmodic for menstrual cramps
- sage, geranium, clary sage, fennel and cypress – to help with the symptoms of the menopause.

# The Immune System

This system is responsible for fighting infection by producing white blood cells and antitoxins. Many essential oils have the property of stimulating the immune function to help the body fight attacks by bacteria and viruses. Treatment is by massage and aromatic baths with the following examples of essential oils:

- lavender, eucalyptus, tea tree, chamomile, pine, and sandalwood – immune stimulating by promoting the formation of white blood cells
- camphor, clove, eucalyptus, tea tree, cajeput, niaouli,

cinnamon, pine, rosemary, bergamot and basil – antibacterial and antiviral.

# The Lymphatic System

The lymphatic system drains and disposes of toxic waste from all parts of the body. It also drains fluids; sluggish lymph circulation results in oedema or fluid retention, especially of the ankles, and cellulite in the thighs, hips and buttocks. Treatment is by massage and compress with the following examples of essential oils:

* fennel, geranium, juniper and rosemary – lymphatic stimulants
* tea tree, thyme, pine, eucalyptus and lemon – antitoxic agents.

# The Nervous System

Most essential oils have both stimulating and sedative effects on the nervous system, although one effect is usually more pronounced than the other, while some have a regulating or balancing effect on the system. Stimulating essential oils are useful for problems such as depression and nervous fatigue; sedative essential oils are useful for problems such as insomnia, nervousness, anxiety and hysteria. Treatment is by massage or aromatic baths with the following examples of essential oils:

* chamomile, melissa, vetivert, lavender, clary sage, neroli, petitgrain, rosewood, rose, jasmine and marjoram – sedative
* cardamon, fennel, cinnamon, basil, clove, anise, peppermint, pine, thyme, rosemary, cajeput, niaouli and camphor – stimulating
* sandalwood, bergamot, geranium, and cedarwood – balancing.

# The Muscular and Skeletal System

Essential oils offer considerable relief to wandering rheumatic stiffness and pain in the muscles and joints by stimulating local circulation and producing warmth. Treatment is by massage or aromatic baths with the following examples of essential oils:

- lavender, rosemary, black pepper and marjoram – for muscle aches
- German chamomile, rosemary, juniper, fennel and celery – for joint stiffness.

# The Skin

The skin covers the whole body, with a total surface area of 1.5 square metres. It protects the body from outside elements and helps to conserve body heat and regulate the elimination of water. Vitamin D is also produced in the skin on exposure to sunlight. The skin can suffer from a state of imbalance resulting in one of four conditions: oiliness, dryness, hydration (too much water) or dehydration (too little water). It can also suffer from injuries, inflammation, infection and unpleasant odours. Essential oils can benefit all these conditions. Treatment is by topical application with the following examples of essential oils:

- lavender, chamomile, geranium, frankincense, myrrh and benzoin – cicatrizing (for healing wounds)
- chamomile, lavender and myrrh – anti-inflammatory
- chamomile, lavender, lemon, pine, thyme, eucalyptus, tea tree, clove, cinnamon, bergamot and lemon – antiseptic (for skin infections)
- bergamot, thyme, juniper, cypress, pine, tea tree, peppermint, lemongrass and citronella – deodorant.

# The Emotions

Essential oils have the ability to affect our emotional responses as well as the physical conditions of our bodies. This is because the limbic system, which is concerned with emotion, is connected to the olfactory nerves in the nose; aromas can therefore evoke immediate and powerful responses in the brain. Inhaling the delicate scents lightly is sufficient to induce an emotional response. The actions of specific essential oils on the mind are described fully in Part 3 (in the section on Recipes for the Emotions).

# ◆ Directory of 60 Essential Oils

angelica seed
aniseed and anise, star
basil
bay
benzoin resinoid
bergamot
black pepper
cajeput
camphor
caraway
cardamon
carrot seed
cedarwood
celery
chamomile, German
chamomile, Maroc
chamomile, Roman
cinnamon leaf
citronella
clary sage
clove leaf
coriander
cumin
cypress
eucalyptus
fennel

frankincense
geranium
ginger
grapefruit
hyssop
jasmine absolute
juniper
lavender
lemon
lemongrass
lime
mandarin
marjoram
melissa
myrrh
neroli (orange flower)
niaouli
nutmeg
orange
palmarosa
parsley
patchouli
peppermint
petitgrain
pine needle
rose

rosemary
rosewood and ho leaf
sage
sandalwood

tea tree
thyme
vetivert
ylang-ylang

The recipes for the conditions listed under each essential oil are to be blended with 25 ml of vegetable oil. The essential oils indicated for emotional conditions can also be used for room vaporization. Each recipe is carefully formulated to correspond to all the problems described under each body system (*see pages 43–9*). The additional essential oils used in each recipe are chosen for their enhancing and balancing effects on the primary oil.

# Angelica

◆ ◇ ◆ ◇ ◆ ◇ ◆ ◇ ◆ ◇ ◆ ◇ ◆ ◇ ◆ ◇ ◆ ◇ ◆ ◇ ◆ ◇ ◆ ◇ ◆ ◇ ◆ ◇ ◆ ◇ ◆ ◇ ◆ ◇

| | |
|---|---|
| **Botanical Name:** | *Angelica archangelica* |
| **Family:** | *Umbelliferae* |
| **Location:** | Cultivated in Belgium, England, Germany, Hungary and Siberia. Also found in Greenland and Iceland. |
| **Extraction:** | Steam distillation of the seeds |
| **Colour and Odour:** | The essential oil is pale yellow in colour and has a sweet, herbaceous and richly musky aroma. |
| **Description:** | A fairly large herb growing quite tall with a hollow stem, large, broad, pointed leaves and greenish-white flowers. Angelica grows near water and can be found along streams and river-banks. The roots can grow to be quite large. |
| **Background:** | Angelica was highly valued in Europe, especially during the Renaissance. The stems have long been prepared as candied slices for decorating cakes and confectionery. It is used to flavour the liqueurs Chartreuse and Benedictine. The plant was named after the Archangel, St Michael. A second essential oil (known as angelica root oil) can also be extracted from the roots. |
| **Properties:** | Tonic, carminative, stimulant, expectorant, diuretic, antispasmodic and emmenagogic. |
| **Precaution:** | The essential oil of angelica root is photo- |

toxic and should not be used shortly before exposure to strong light. However, the oil obtained from the seeds is not phototoxic.

Uses:   DIGESTIVE SYSTEM – Stimulates appetite and is beneficial for anorexia nervosa.
URINARY SYSTEM – Promotes kidney function and helps with all types of problems affecting urine flow.
CIRCULATORY SYSTEM – Tonic to the heart and promotes circulation. Good for anaemia.
RESPIRATORY SYSTEM – Angelica's expectorant property is helpful for chronic bronchitis and pleurisy.
REPRODUCTIVE SYSTEM – Promotes menstrual flow and is useful for period problems.
EMOTION – Revitalizes a fatigued mind and loss of interest in life; also relieves impatience and exhaustion. Promotes courage in the emotionally weak. Good for those with an indifferent attitude.

## Blends:

**DIGESTIVE:**
| angelica | 6 |
| coriander | 5 |
| cardamon | 2 |

**URINARY:**
| angelica | 6 |
| celery | 4 |
| rosmary | 3 |

**CIRCULATORY:**
| angelica | 6 |
| rosemary | 5 |
| melissa | 2 |

**RESPIRATORY:**
| angelica | 5 |
| benzoin | 4 |
| pine | 3 |

**REPRODUCTIVE:**
| angelica | 5 |
| rose | 4 |
| marjoram | 3 |

**EMOTION:**
| angelica | 4 |
| mandarin | 3 |
| sandalwood | 2 |

# Aniseed and Anise, Star

| | |
|---|---|
| **Botanical Name:** | *Pimpinella anisum* and *Illicium verum* |
| **Family:** | *Umbelliferae* and *Illiciaceae* |
| **Location:** | Aniseed is found in Egypt, Greece, Spain and India; anise, star is found in southeast China and Vietnam. |
| **Extraction:** | Steam distillation of the seeds. |
| **Colour and Odour:** | Both of these essential oils are clear with a hint of yellow. They have a very anisic aroma with sweet undertones. |
| **Description:** | Aniseed is a small herb growing to about 60 cm with bright green delicate leaves and tiny white flowers. Anise, star is an evergreen tree growing up to about 9 m with a slender white trunk, yellow flowers and star-shaped fruits. |
| **Background:** | The essential oils of these two plants have very similar chemical compositions and medicinal properties. They are listed in the pharmacopoeias as acceptable substitutes for each other. Their aromas are virtually identical and they are used in the same way in aromatherapy. |
| | Aniseed was known to the ancient Egyptians and used by them in bread-making; the Greeks and Romans followed suit and aniseed is still used for this purpose in Europe. Anise, star has long been used by the Chinese in cooking and medicine. |

An important use of both aniseed and anise, star is as a corrector to unpleasant medicines.

Properties: Stimulant, expectorant, diuretic, antispasmodic and tonic.

Precaution: This oil is best used in lower concentrations as it may cause irritation in sensitive people and may be over-stimulating.

Uses: DIGESTIVE SYSTEM – Helpful for flatulent colic and the gripe-like pains of indigestion.
URINARY SYSTEM – Promotes the flow of urine.
RESPIRATORY SYSTEM – Very useful for respiratory problems including bronchitis, and also spasmodic problems such as dry irritable coughs and whooping cough.
REPRODUCTIVE SYSTEM – Calms menstrual cramps.
EMOTION – Invigorates a tired mind.

**Blends:**

| DIGESTIVE: | | URINARY: | | RESPIRATORY: | |
|---|---|---|---|---|---|
| anise | 5 | anise | 5 | anise | 5 |
| rosemary | 3 | cypress | 4 | myrrh | 4 |
| cardamon | 3 | parsley | 2 | pine | 3 |

| REPRODUCTIVE: | | EMOTION: | |
|---|---|---|---|
| anise | 5 | anise | 5 |
| chamomile (R) | 4 | orange | 4 |
| geranium | 2 | lime | 3 |

# Basil

◆◇◆◇◆◇◆◇◆◇◆◇◆◇◆◇◆◇◆◇◆◇◆◇◆◇◆◇◆◇◆◇◆◇

| | |
|---|---|
| **Botanical Name:** | *Ocimum basilicum* |
| **Family:** | *Labiatae* |
| **Location:** | Basil is found in tropical Africa and India. It is now cultivated in the Comoro Islands, Egypt, France and Madagascar. |
| **Extraction:** | Steam distillation of the leaves. |
| **Colour and Odour:** | The essential oil is colourless, having a very pleasant, rich, refreshing, sweet, spicy, green and piercing odour. |
| **Description:** | A delicate plant growing up to 90 cm in height with light-green oval leaves and white flowers. |
| **Background:** | The name is derived from the Greek 'basilicon', meaning royal. Basil has a long history of use in India, where it is known as 'tulsi' and is held to be sacred to the Hindu gods Krishna and Vishnu. |
| **Properties:** | Stimulating, uplifting, clarifying, strengthening, antiseptic, expectorant, antispasmodic and nervine. |
| **Precaution:** | This oil is best used in lower concentrations as it may cause irritation in sensitive people. |

**Uses:**   DIGESTIVE SYSTEM – Eases vomiting, abdominal cramps and swelling caused by indigestion and flatulence.

RESPIRATORY SYSTEM – Useful for sinus

congestion, asthma, bronchitis and emphysema.
Basil is also recommended for chronic colds and
influenza as well as hiccups and whooping cough.

REPRODUCTIVE SYSTEM – Will assist painful and/or
scanty periods.

NERVOUS SYSTEM – An excellent nerve tonic,
basil is useful for all types of nervous disorders,
especially those associated with weakness,
indecision or hysteria. Also valuable for states of
nervousness, anxiety and depression.

MUSCULAR SYSTEM – Basil is very good for tired or
overworked muscles, especially after strenuous
physical exercise. It strengthens tense or flaccid
muscles.

EMOTION – Basil clears the head, strengthens the
memory, aids concentration, sharpens the intellect,
relieves mental fatigue and is helpful during times
of mental effort, promoting alertness in the
morning and sound sleep at night.

## Blends:

| DIGESTIVE: | | RESPIRATORY: | | REPRODUCTIVE: | |
|---|---|---|---|---|---|
| basil | 5 | basil | 6 | basil | 5 |
| peppermint | 3 | pine | 3 | lavender | 4 |
| chamomile (R) | 3 | benzoin | 3 | jasmine | 3 |

| NERVOUS: | | MUSCULAR: | | EMOTION: | |
|---|---|---|---|---|---|
| basil | 5 | basil | 6 | basil | 4 |
| lavender | 3 | marjoram | 4 | lemon | 4 |
| chamomile (R) | 3 | rosemary | 3 | juniper | 4 |

# Bay

◆ ◇ ◆ ^ ◆ ◇ ◆ ◇ ◆ ^ ◆ ◇ ◆ ◇ ◆ ◇ ◆ ◇ ◆ ◇ ◆ ◇ ◆ ◇ ◆ ◇ ◆ ◇ ◆ ◇ ◆ ◇ ◆ ◇ ◆ ◇

| | |
|---|---|
| **Botanical Name:** | *Pimenta racemosa* |
| **Family:** | *Myrtaceae* |
| **Location:** | Bay is found in Dominica, Jamaica and Mexico. |
| **Extraction:** | Steam distillation of the leaves. |
| **Colour and Odour:** | The essential oil is dark brown in colour with a strong, warm and spicy aroma. |
| **Description:** | A wild growing, sturdy, evergreen tropical tree growing up to 9 m. It has large, leathery leaves and aromatic fruits. The trees are particularly abundant in Dominica. |
| **Background:** | The bay tree is often grown in groves together with the allspice bush. The fruits of both are dried and powdered for use as spices. Bay leaves are used in Jamaica for flavouring West Indian Bay Rum, which is a famous hair tonic used especially for a greasy scalp. |
| **Properties:** | Stimulant, antiseptic, tonic, expectorant, analgesic, anticonvulsant, antineuralgic, antirheumatic and astringent. |

Uses:   RESPIRATORY SYSTEM – Bay's antiseptic quality is
        useful in bronchitis, colds and flu.
        SKIN – A good tonic for the hair and scalp, bay
        stimulates hair growth and also helps to clear
        dandruff.
        EMOTION – Bay is slightly euphoric, lifting the
        spirits. It stimulates imaginative decisions, is
        distinctive and inspires confidence. Promotes
        courage in the submissive.

## Blends:

| RESPIRATORY: | | SKIN: | | EMOTION: | |
|---|---|---|---|---|---|
| bay | 5 | bay | 5 | bay | 5 |
| benzoin | 4 | cedarwood | 5 | grapefruit | 4 |
| eucalyptus | 3 | rosemary | 3 | ginger | 2 |

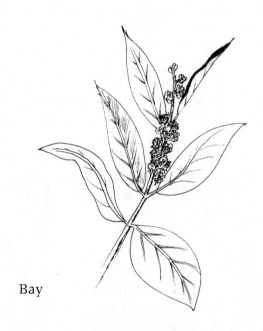

Bay

# Benzoin (Resinoid)

◆◇◆◇◆◇◆◇◆◇◆◇◆◇◆◇◆◇◆◇◆◇◆◇◆◇◆◇◆◇◆◇

| | |
|---|---|
| **Botanical Name:** | *Styrax benzoin* |
| **Family:** | *Styracaceae* |
| **Location:** | Benzoin is found in Cambodia, Java, Laos, Sumatra, Thailand and Vietnam. |
| **Extraction:** | Solvent extraction of the gum. |
| **Colour and Odour:** | Benzoin resinoid is thick and dark golden-brown in colour, having a most pleasant aroma resembling vanilla. It is one of the heavier oils and is an excellent fixative. |
| **Description:** | The benzoin tree grows in tropical Asia, where it is also cultivated. The natural gum is collected from deep incisions made in the tree trunk; it hardens on exposure to the air. |
| **Background:** | Long used in antiquity as an incense. Known in Europe during the Middle Ages when it was used as a compound tincture for inhalation. It was then called 'Friar's Balsam'. |
| **Note:** | Benzoin is a resinoid and cannot be obtained as a pure essential oil. The resinoid is the natural extract from the tree, which is then diluted with a solvent (benzyl alcohol). This makes it easier to pour and handle, as the natural product is very thick and difficult to use. |
| **Properties:** | Warming, energizing, circulatory stimulant,sedative, decongesting, expectorant, diuretic, carminative. |

**Uses:**    URINARY SYSTEM – Antiseptic property good for cystitis.

RESPIRATORY SYSTEM – Tonic to the lungs. Effective for colds, flu, bronchitis and asthma, clearing and expelling congested mucus. Also good for coughs, sore throat and loss of voice.

REPRODUCTIVE SYSTEM – Excellent for leucorrhoea.

MUSCULAR SYSTEM – Good for rheumatism.

SKIN – Soothing for conditions where there is redness, irritation and itching, such as cracked skin or chapped hands, chilblains and dermatitis. A good remedy for wounds and sores.

EMOTION – Calming and comforting for crisis states involving sadness, loneliness, depression and anxiety. Especially good for dispelling anger. In times of great exertion, benzoin eases emotional exhaustion, is energizing and increases physical strength. The scent of benzoin stimulates the conscious mind and counteracts indifference. Benzoin is protective against life's crises. It also releases past tensions and resentments.

## Blends:

| URINARY: | | RESPIRATORY: | | REPRODUCTIVE: | |
|---|---|---|---|---|---|
| benzoin | 7 | benzoin | 6 | benzoin | 6 |
| celery | 4 | eucalyptus | 5 | sandalwood | 3 |
| niaouli | 2 | thyme | 3 | bergamot | 3 |

| MUSCULAR: | | SKIN: | | EMOTION: | |
|---|---|---|---|---|---|
| benzoin | 7 | benzoin | 5 | benzoin | 6 |
| marjoram | 4 | myrrh | 2 | rose | 4 |
| juniper | 3 | chamomile (R) | 2 | clary sage | 2 |

61

# Bergamot

◆ ◇ ◆ ◇ ◆ ◇ ◆ ◇ ◆ ◇ ◆ ◇ ◆ ◇ ◆ ◇ ◆ ◇ ◆ ◇ ◆ ◇ ◆ ◇ ◆ ◇ ◆ ◇ ◆ ◇ ◆ ◇ ◆ ◇ ◆ ◇

| | |
|---|---|
| **Botanical Name:** | *Citrus bergamia* |
| **Family:** | *Rutaceae* |
| **Location:** | Bergamot is cultivated in the Ivory Coast, southern Italy and Sicily. |
| **Extraction:** | Expression of the ripe fruit peel. |
| **Colour and Odour:** | The essential oil is a green colour and has a citrusy and sweet aroma with a light, delicate floral hint. |
| **Description:** | The bergamot tree bears fruits resembling oranges which are slightly pear-shaped. |
| **Background:** | The bergamot fruit was developed for its scent, which has been used in perfumery since the eighteenth century. It was named after the city of Bergamo in the northern Italian district of Lombardy. It has been used in Italian folk medicine for many years. Bergamot is used to flavour Earl Grey tea; the essential oil is an ingredient of Eau-de-Cologne. |
| **Properties:** | Antispasmodic, carminative, antiseptic, sedative and uplifting. |
| **Precaution:** | Bergamot essential oil is phototoxic. Do not use before being exposed to strong UV light. |

**Uses:**  DIGESTIVE SYSTEM – Bergamot will stimulate appetite in cases of anorexia nervosa, and will also help to regulate the appetite of compulsive eaters.

URINARY SYSTEM – Strongly indicated for all urinary tract infections including cystitis and urethritis.

REPRODUCTIVE SYSTEM – Effective for vaginal pruritus and leucorrhoea.

SKIN – Useful in treating oily skin, boils and acne. Also effective for cold sores.

EMOTION – Bergamot's uplifting and balancing qualities are very useful for treating listlessness, depression and anxiety. It can encourage a restful, relaxing sleep at night. Its sharp, keen scent helps to instil confidence and aids in the recouping of emotional control by helping the individual let go and open up.

## Blends:

**DIGESTIVE:**

| | |
|---|---|
| bergamot | 7 |
| anise | 3 |
| ginger | 2 |

**URINARY:**

| | |
|---|---|
| bergamot | 7 |
| juniper | 4 |
| sandalwood | 3 |

**REPRODUCTIVE:**

| | |
|---|---|
| bergamot | 4 |
| myrrh | 4 |
| chamomile (R) | 3 |

**SKIN:**

| | |
|---|---|
| bergamot | 6 |
| lavender | 4 |
| tea tree | 3 |

**EMOTION:**

| | |
|---|---|
| bergamot | 8 |
| cypress | 3 |
| lavender | 2 |

# Black Pepper

| | |
|---|---|
| **Botanical Name:** | *Piper nigrum* |
| **Family:** | *Piperaceae* |
| **Location:** | Pepper is cultivated mainly in India and Malaysia. |
| **Extraction:** | Steam distillation of the ripe peppercorns. |
| **Colour and Odour:** | The essential oil is colourless with a strong, penetrating, sharp and spicy middle note and an unexpectedly refined, warm aroma quite unlike the spice itself. |
| **Description:** | A climbing vine with dark green leaves, white flowers and red berries, growing to about 6 m. Originally a forest plant, now widely cultivated on supports reaching up to a maximum of 3.5 m for convenience. The spice is available as white or black pepper, but the essential oil is obtained from black pepper. |
| **Background:** | Pepper is probably the earliest known spice and was highly regarded and prized. It was very popular with both the Romans and the Greeks. Later the European powers fought over its monopoly, the Portuguese and Dutch having the most influence over the spice islands of the East. As a spice, pepper is among the most important in the world. |
| **Properties:** | Warming, rubefacient, circulatory stimulant, expectorant, antispasmodic, |

carminative, aphrodisiac and tonic.

**Precaution:** This oil is best used in lower concentrations as it may cause irritation in sensitive people.

**Uses:** DIGESTIVE SYSTEM – Valuable for dyspepsia and sluggish digestion. Pepper's antispasmodic action soothes the gut and restores tone to lax muscles of the colon. Helps to ease the constipation caused by colds and cold weather conditions. Also good for loss of appetite. Acts as an antitoxic agent in food poisoning.

URINARY SYSTEM – Stimulates the kidneys and can be used as a diuretic.

CIRCULATORY SYSTEM – Pepper's ability to increase the circulation (like ginger) makes it helpful for people with cold limbs. It is indicated where there is extreme physical or emotional cold. It is a spleen tonic. Useful for anaemia and bruising.

RESPIRATORY SYSTEM – Good remedy for colds and flu. The warming and expectorant action on the respiratory system promptly clears mucus. It brings on a sweat and can be helpful in the first shivery stages of a cold or flu.

MUSCULAR SYSTEM: Pepper is good for rheumatic pains.

EMOTION – Pepper has cephalic qualities, stimulating and strengthening the nerves and the mind. It is helpful for indifference and frustration or hidden angers, offering stamina and strength. Pepper helps with alertness and concentration, especially for individuals who tend to daydream or drowse during meditation or long-distance driving. It is also useful for bolstering courage in stressful situations such as public speaking or confronting a difficult person.

## Blends:

| DIGESTIVE: | | URINARY: | | CIRCULATORY: | |
|---|---|---|---|---|---|
| B pepper | 6 | B pepper | 7 | B pepper | 6 |
| marjoram | 3 | fennel | 3 | marjoram | 3 |
| anise | 2 | parsley | 2 | rosemary | 3 |

| RESPIRATORY: | | MUSCULAR: | | EMOTION: | |
|---|---|---|---|---|---|
| B pepper | 6 | B pepper | 6 | B pepper | 5 |
| benzoin | 4 | coriander | 4 | lemon | 4 |
| pine | 2 | lavender | 3 | cedarwood | 3 |

This is a particularly interesting essence. It has its own personality and past. In Greece the plant was used against intermittent fever which was in actual fact a mild form of Mediterranean malaria. It was also believed to fortify the stomach. The mendicant monks of India who cover daily considerable distances on foot, swallow seven to nine grains of pepper a day. This gives them remarkable endurance.

Experience has taught us that the essential oil of pepper exerts a great influence on the muscular tonus; it seems that here we have the reason why the pepper acts on the contractions of the stomach which, as everyone knows, is a muscle. We often use it in the case of muscular atonia.

*Marguerite Maury*

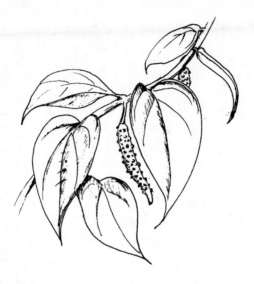

Black Pepper

# Cajeput

◆◇◆◇◆◇◆◇◆◇◆◇◆◇◆◇◆◇◆◇◆◇◆◇◆◇◆◇◆◇◆◇◆◇◆◇◆◇◆◇

| | |
|---|---|
| **Botanical Name:** | *Melaleuca leucadendron* |
| **Family:** | *Myrtaceae* |
| **Location:** | Cajeput is found in Australia, Indonesia, Malaysia and the Philippines. |
| **Extraction:** | Steam distillation of the leaves. |
| **Colour and Odour:** | The essential oil is clear with a hint of yellow; it has a penetrating, camphorous aroma. |
| **Description:** | A tree with a whitish bark growing up to 13.5 m. The bark is fibrous and loose, coming off naturally in large strips. Growth is vigorous and spontaneous; regrowth occurs if the bark is destroyed, so cultivation is minimal. |
| **Background:** | Valued by the Malays, Chinese and Indians for its medicinal properties. The leaves are used locally for respiratory and muscular problems. However, in Europe only the oil is used, in herbal medicines for its warming qualities. First introduced during the seventeenth century, the Dutch seem to have been the first Europeans to have used it, although later the French also found it useful. |
| **Properties:** | Antiseptic, expectorant, stimulant, tonic, analgesic, antispasmodic. |

**Uses:** RESPIRATORY SYSTEM – Eases chronic pulmonary problems. Good for colds, flu and sinusitis.

MUSCULAR SYSTEM – Useful for general stiffness, sore muscles, rheumatism and general weakness and fatigue.

EMOTION – Stimulating for the mind, good for mental fatigue, apathy and cynicism. Also helpful for a state of disorientation and a tendency to procrastination.

## Blends:

| RESPIRATORY: | | MUSCULAR: | | EMOTION: | |
| --- | --- | --- | --- | --- | --- |
| cajeput | 6 | cajeput | 6 | cajeput | 5 |
| pine | 4 | rosemary | 3 | lemon | 4 |
| lavender | 2 | marjoram | 3 | eucalyptus | 3 |

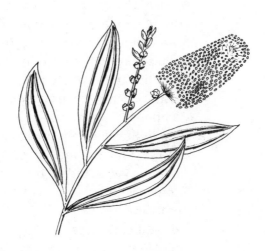

Cajeput

# Camphor

◆ ♢ ◆ ♢ ◆ ♢ ◆ ♢ ◆ ♢ ◆ ♢ ◆ ♢ ◆ ♢ ◆ ♢ ◆ ♢ ◆ ♢ ◆ ♢ ◆ ♢ ◆ ♢ ◆ ♢ ◆ ♢ ◆ ♢

| | |
|---|---|
| **Botanical Name:** | *Cinnamomum camphora* |
| **Family:** | *Lauraceae* |
| **Location:** | Camphor trees are found in China, Japan and Taiwan. |
| **Extraction:** | Steam distillation of the crude camphor obtained by boiling the wood in water. |
| **Colour and Odour:** | The essential oil is colourless with a fresh and pungent aroma. |
| **Description:** | Camphor trees are hardy evergreen trees growing up to 30 m tall. The trees have straight trunks with small leaves, white flowers occurring in clusters and dark red berries. The camphor is formed in white crystalline masses of about 25–30 cm, found mainly in the trunks of mature trees but also present in every part of the tree. |
| **Background:** | Camphor trees were planted in Taoist and Buddhist temples throughout China. Camphor was also valued in India. It was used in Europe from the late seventeenth century. The therapeutic properties of camphor were studied thoroughly by Samuel Hahnemann, the founder of homoeopathy. |
| **Properties:** | Antiseptic, analgesic, respiratory and circulatory tonic, stimulant, nerve sedative, antispasmodic, anti-inflammatory and rubefacient. |

Uses:    RESPIRATORY SYSTEM – Stimulates respiration,
         clears congested lungs and eases breathing. It also
         speeds recovery from colds.
         MUSCULAR SYSTEM – Helpful with stiff muscles
         and eases rheumatic aches and pains.
         EMOTION – Camphor has a very balancing effect,
         dispelling apathy and daydreaming. Lessens
         strong sexual urges.

**Blends:**

| RESPIRATORY: | | MUSCULAR: | | EMOTION: | |
|---|---|---|---|---|---|
| camphor | 6 | camphor | 6 | camphor | 5 |
| pine | 3 | ginger | 4 | bergamot | 3 |
| myrrh | 3 | coriander | 3 | chamomile (M) | 2 |

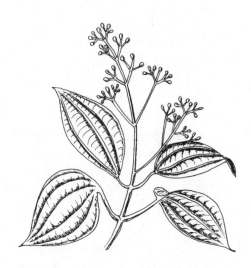

Camphor

# Caraway

| | |
|---|---|
| Botanical Name: | *Carum carvi* |
| Family: | *Umbelliferae* |
| Location: | Caraway is found in Europe and western Asia. It is cultivated in Germany, Holland, Russia and Scandinavia. |
| Extraction: | Steam distillation of the seeds. |
| Colour and Odour: | The essential oil is pale yellow in colour and has a sweet, sharp, slightly spicy aroma. |
| Description: | A small herb growing to 60 cm with green stalks, feathery leaves and tufted, pinkish-white flowers. |
| Background: | Known to the ancient Egyptians, Greeks and Romans. The seeds are popular in Arab and northern European countries as a flavouring in baking and pastries, especially in rye breads. Caraway is also a main ingredient of the German liqueur, 'Kummel'. |
| Properties: | Carminative, digestive, diuretic, antispasmodic, antiseptic, stimulant and tonic. |

Uses:  DIGESTIVE SYSTEM – Tonic to the digestive tract. Helps with indigestion by stimulating the intestinal walls and easing the spasms caused by flatulence. URINARY SYSTEM – Promotes the flow of urine and encourages the flushing of toxins.

REPRODUCTIVE SYSTEM – Promotes menstruation and also milk flow.

SKIN – Effective in tissue regeneration, helping with bruises. Also useful for skin problems such as acne, boils and scabies.

EMOTION – Stimulating and refreshing to the mind, caraway enhances alertness and strengthens the memory. It eases mental strain and fatigue, replenishing lost energy.

## Blends:

| DIGESTIVE: | | URINARY: | | REPRODUCTIVE: | |
|---|---|---|---|---|---|
| caraway | 6 | caraway | 6 | caraway | 5 |
| B pepper | 4 | juniper | 4 | fennel | 3 |
| ginger | 2 | rosemary | 3 | rosemary | 2 |

| SKIN: | | EMOTION: | |
|---|---|---|---|
| caraway | 5 | caraway | 5 |
| chamomile (R) | 4 | palmarosa | 4 |
| lemon | 3 | basil | 3 |

# Cardamon

◆ ◇ ◆ ^ ◆ ◡ ◆ ◡ ◆ ^ ◆ ◡ ◆ ◡ ◆ ◇ ◆ ◡ ◆ ◡ ◆ ◇ ◆ ◡ ◆ ◇ ◆ ◇ ◆ ◇ ◆ ◡ ◆ ◇ ◆ ◡ ◆ ◇ ◆ ◇ ◆ ◇ ◆

| | |
|---|---|
| **Botanical Name:** | *Elettaria cardamomum* |
| **Family:** | *Zingiberaceae* |
| **Location:** | Cardamon is cultivated mainly in India and Sri Lanka. |
| **Extraction:** | Steam distillation of the seeds. |
| **Colour and Odour:** | The essential oil is pale yellow with an agreeable, warm, sweet and spicy aroma. |
| **Description:** | A leafy stemmed shrub with very long leaves from 30–75 cm long and pale yellow flowers. The fruits are oval and greyish in colour, about 1.25 cm long, and contain dark brown seeds. |
| **Background:** | Cardamon has a long history of use in India. Also known to the ancient Egyptians and used by the Greeks and the Romans. The Arabs later also recognized its digestive properties, often grinding it with their coffee. Cardamon is popular in Eastern European countries. |
| **Properties:** | Warming, tonic, stimulant, refreshing, invigorating, digestive and aphrodisiac. |

**Uses:**   DIGESTIVE SYSTEM – A digestive aid, cardamon corrects indigestion and gastric fermentation. It is good for flatulence and freshens the breath. Cardamon is mainly recommended for chronic indigestion with bloating, belching, flatulence and hiccups. It is an effective remedy for heartburn as it relieves pressure in the chest caused by a swollen stomach pressing on the diaphragm.

URINARY SYSTEM – As a diuretic, cardamon remedies urine retention.

EMOTION – Cardamon's distinct, uplifting and lightening effect helps to clear the mind of confusion. Cheers the heart and counters selfishness. Stimulates the mind to enable clear thinking.

## Blends:

| DIGESTIVE: | | URINARY: | | EMOTION: | |
|---|---|---|---|---|---|
| cardamon | 5 | cardamon | 5 | cardamon | 5 |
| ginger | 3 | celery | 4 | basil | 3 |
| parsley | 3 | fennel | 3 | lemon | 3 |

# Carrot Seed

◆ ◇ ◆ ◇ ◆ ◇ ◆ ◇ ◆ ◇ ◆ ◇ ◆ ◇ ◆ ◇ ◆ ◇ ◆ ◇ ◆ ◇ ◆ ◇ ◆ ◇ ◆ ◇ ◆ ◇ ◆ ◇ ◆ ◇ ◆ ◇

| | |
|---|---|
| **Botanical Name:** | *Daucus carota* |
| **Family:** | *Umbelliferae* |
| **Location:** | The wild carrot is found in Europe, India and North Africa. The essential oil is distilled in France. |
| **Extraction:** | Steam distillation of the seeds. |
| **Colour and Odour:** | The essential oil is clear with a hint of yellow; it has a herby, woody and earthy aroma. |
| **Description:** | The essential oil is obtained from the seeds of the wild carrot, which have a stringy tap root unlike the thick succulent root of the more familiar cultivated carrot. Both the wild and cultivated carrots are herbs with green stalks and leaves and white lacy flower tops with purple centres. |
| **Background:** | The carrot has long been cultivated for its fleshy bright orange tap root. It is important for its vitamin A content, which is good for the eyesight. Another beneficial oil can also extracted from the carrot roots. |
| **Properties:** | Tonic, carminative, diuretic, hepatic, emmenagogic, cytophylactic and stimulant. |

**Uses:** DIGESTIVE SYSTEM – Carrot has a tonic action on the liver and gall-bladder and is used for treating jaundice.

URINARY SYSTEM – Promotes urine flow; beneficial
for cystitis.

REPRODUCTIVE SYSTEM – Promotes menstruation,
useful for absent or scanty periods. Also good for
menstrual cramps.

SKIN – Restores tone and elasticity to skin and
helps to reduce wrinkles. Good for blemished skin
and will benefit both dry and oily skin types.
Carrot improves the complexion and confers a
more youthful appearance.

EMOTION – Strengthens the mind and helps
with doubt and confusion. Also useful for over-
excitability and nervousness.

## Blends:

| DIGESTIVE: | | | URINARY: | | | REPRODUCTIVE: | |
|---|---|---|---|---|---|---|---|
| carrot | 5 | | carrot | 5 | | carrot | 6 |
| cardamon | 4 | | juniper | 4 | | juniper | 4 |
| ginger | 3 | | sandalwood | 3 | | geranium | 3 |

| SKIN: | | | EMOTION: | |
|---|---|---|---|---|
| carrot | 3 | | carrot | 4 |
| frankincense | 2 | | rosewood | 4 |
| neroli | 2 | | orange | 3 |

# Cedarwood

◆ ◇ ◆ ◇ ◆ ◇ ◆ ◇ ◆ ◇ ◆ ◇ ◆ ◇ ◆ ◇ ◆ ◇ ◆ ◇ ◆ ◇ ◆ ◇ ◆ ◇ ◆ ◇ ◆ ◇ ◆ ◇ ◆ ◇

**Botanical Name:** *Cedrus atlantica*

**Family:** *Pinaceae*

**Location:** The Atlas cedar is found in the Atlas Mountains of Morocco and Algeria. The Cedar of Lebanon, closely related to the Atlas cedar, grows in the Middle East where, sadly, great forests have been reduced to small groves due to over-exploitation.

**Extraction:** Steam distillation of the wood chips.

**Colour and Odour:** The essential oil is yellow in colour and viscid, resembling sandalwood. It has a rich, warm, woody and masculine fragrance which is harmonious and long lasting.

**Description:** A stately evergreen tree growing up to 40 m high. The wood is hard and highly aromatic.

**Background:** The Cedar of Lebanon has been used since ancient times as incense and also for timber in Egypt. Solomon bought vast quantities to build the Great Temple in Jerusalem during biblical times. Also used by Tibetan monks as a temple incense to aid meditation.

**Properties:** Sedative, astringent, expectorant, tonic, antiseptic and mucolytic.

Uses:    URINARY SYSTEM – Good for painful or difficult
         urination. A valuable remedy for cystitis with
         burning pain.
         SKIN – Valuable for all types of skin eruptions;
         relieves itching. Very good for oily hair and
         dandruff.
         EMOTION – Cedarwood clears the mind when it is
         clogged with anxiety and nervous tension. Good
         for daydreamers and the absent-minded. It releases
         aggression and relaxes the analytical mind. Helps
         individuals to develop a sense of balance and self-
         control in their lives. Cedarwood gives strength
         and fortitude, creates harmony and encourages
         sexual response.

**Blends:**

| URINARY: | | SKIN: | | EMOTION: | |
|---|---|---|---|---|---|
| cedarwood | 7 | cedarwood | 6 | cedarwood | 6 |
| lavender | 3 | chamomile (R) | 3 | geranium | 2 |
| juniper | 2 | mandarin | 2 | lemon | 2 |

# Celery

◆ ◇ ◆ ◇ ◆ ◇ ◆ ◇ ◆ ◇ ◆ ◇ ◆ ◇ ◆ ◇ ◆ ◇ ◆ ◇ ◆ ◇ ◆ ◇ ◆ ◇ ◆ ◇ ◆ ◇ ◆ ◇ ◆ ◇ ◆ ◇

| | |
|---|---|
| **Botanical Name:** | *Apium graveolens* |
| **Family:** | *Umbelliferae* |
| **Location:** | Celery grows in southern Europe. The essential oil is obtained from plants cultivated in Holland, Hungary and India. |
| **Extraction:** | Distillation of the seeds. |
| **Colour and Odour:** | The essential oil is pale yellow in colour with a fresh, warm, sweet-spicy aroma. |
| **Description:** | A small herb with fleshy erect stalks about 60 cm high having light green, delicate leaves and whitish flowers. |
| **Background:** | Celery was known to the ancient Greeks and was later used by Western Europeans as a cultivated vegetable. Another variety of celery is the celeriac root vegetable. |
| **Properties:** | Carminative, diuretic, sedative, hypotensive, tonic, and antirheumatic. |

**Uses:** DIGESTIVE SYSTEM – Useful in expelling wind and relieving a bloated stomach.

URINARY SYSTEM – Promotes the flow of urine; clears the body of toxins. Decreases puffiness due to water retention. It is also antiseptic, thereby good for combating cystitis.

CIRCULATORY SYSTEM – Helpful for high blood pressure.

REPRODUCTIVE SYSTEM – Helpful in menstrual problems, as it clears obstructions.

SKELETAL SYSTEM – Dissolves toxic accumulations in the joints, relieving rheumatic and arthritic problems.

EMOTION – Helps to induce cheerfulness after a tiring day. Clears mental clutter and reduces anxiety.

## Blends:

| DIGESTIVE: | | URINARY: | | CIRCULATORY: | |
|---|---|---|---|---|---|
| celery | 6 | celery | 6 | celery | 6 |
| melissa | 4 | juniper | 5 | rose | 3 |
| peppermint | 2 | rosemary | 2 | ylang-ylang | 2 |

| REPRODUCTIVE: | | SKELETAL: | | EMOTION: | |
|---|---|---|---|---|---|
| celery | 6 | celery | 7 | celery | 6 |
| rosemary | 4 | rosemary | 3 | rosewood | 3 |
| rose | 3 | marjoram | 3 | orange | 2 |

# Chamomiles

Botanical Names:     *Anthemis nobilis* (Roman chamomile);
    *Matricaria chamomilla* (German chamomile);
    *Ormenis multicaulis* (Maroc chamomile)

Family:     *Compositae*

Location:     Roman chamomile is found in Belgium, England, France and Italy; German chamomile is cultivated in Hungary; Maroc chamomile is found in northwest Africa, Spain and Israel.

Extraction:     Steam distillation of the flowers.

Colour and Odour:     The German and Roman chamomiles are blue in colour, while the chamomile Maroc is pale yellow. With age the Roman chamomile turns from a very pale blue to colourless. However, this change does not affect the therapeutic quality of the oil. The German chamomile remains a deep blue. The blue colour of the essential oils is due to their azulene content, which is most present in the German chamomile oil. (Azulene is responsible for the anti-inflammatory properties of chamomile oils.) These three essential oils have a rich, warm, distinctive fruity smell, with undertones reminiscent of over-ripe apples.

Description:     There are three plants called 'chamomile' having essential oils of similar aroma and therapeutic qualities. They are all strongly aromatic, herbaceous plants with daisy-like, yellow flowers.

**Background:** The Roman and German chamomiles have a long tradition of herbal use in Europe brewed as a tea for both internal and external use. Maroc chamomile oil is a more recent introduction. It contains less azulene than the other two and is becoming popular because it is the most reasonably priced of the three. Roman chamomile is a popular lawn plant as its scent becomes more noticeable when it is walked on.

**Properties:** Stomachic, hepatic, nervine, emollient, carminative, stimulant, antispasmodic, sedative, diuretic, antidepressant, antiphlogistic, anti-allergenic, anti-inflammatory, analgesic and antiseptic.

**Uses:** DIGESTIVE SYSTEM: Improves the appetite, and aids atonic dyspepsia by increasing the digestive action. Relieves the vomiting caused by gastritis and heartburn.

URINARY SYSTEM: Relieves renal inflammation and cystitis. Promotes the flow of urine and will also reduce fluid retention.

REPRODUCTIVE SYSTEM: Good for many disorders including scanty, painful or irregular menstruation and menopausal problems. Chamomile is soothing for sore nipples.

NERVOUS SYSTEM: Diminishes nervous excitability and used as a remedy for hysterical and nervous afflictions. Soothes neuralgic pain.

MUSCULAR SYSTEM: Good for general muscular aches and pains.

SKELETAL SYSTEM: Beneficial for painful arthritic joints.

SKIN: Good for dry, sensitive or red skin; useful for skin eruptions such as dermatitis, eczema, psoriasis, acne or rashes and the itching caused by allergies. Also an excellent remedy for inflamed wounds, sores, scarring and burns.

EMOTION: For over-sensitivity, restlessness, nervous irritability, depression, impatience, and all states of anger and agitation. Chamomile dispels emotional distress from the past, tension and fear, and aids emotional stability, freeing the mind from worry. Chamomile is relaxing and helps with insomnia, promoting peaceful sleep.

CHILDREN: Chamomile is a safe remedy for all sorts of children's problems such as colic, diarrhoea, convulsions and even tantrums.

## Blends:

| DIGESTIVE: | | URINARY: | | REPRODUCTIVE: | |
|---|---|---|---|---|---|
| chamomile (R) | 7 | chamomile (G) | 6 | chamomile (R) | 5 |
| ginger | 4 | juniper | 5 | rose | 4 |
| cardamon | 2 | sandalwood | 2 | geranium | 2 |

| NERVOUS: | | MUSCULAR: | | SKELETAL: | |
|---|---|---|---|---|---|
| chamomile (R) | 7 | chamomile (R) | 5 | chamomile (G) | 4 |
| lavender | 3 | lavender | 4 | juniper | 4 |
| rose | 3 | marjoram | 3 | rosemary | 4 |

| SKIN: | | EMOTION: | | CHILDREN: | |
|---|---|---|---|---|---|
| chamomile (R) | 4 | chamomile (M) | 5 | chamomile (R) | 2 |
| lavender | 2 | orange | 4 | lavender | 2 |
| myrrh | 2 | cedarwood | 3 | mandarin | 2 |

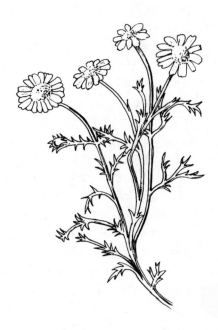

Chamomile

# Cinnamon

◆◇◆◇◆◇◆◇◆◇◆◇◆◇◆◇◆◇◆◇◆◇◆◇◆◇◆◇◆◇◆◇◆◇

| | |
|---|---|
| **Botanical Name:** | *Cinnamomum zeylanicum* |
| **Family:** | *Lauraceae* |
| **Location:** | Cinnamon is cultivated in Comores, India, Madagascar, Seychelles and Sri Lanka. |
| **Extraction:** | Steam distillation of the leaves. |
| **Colour and Odour:** | The essential oil is yellow in colour and has a hot, sharp, spicy odour with a slightly sweet undertone. |
| **Description:** | An evergreen tropical tree growing up to 9 m. It is cultivated for the inner bark, which is collected and dried and later sold as cinnamon spice in the form of squills. The leaves and bark are also distilled to produce leaf and bark essential oils. The leaf essential oil is preferred for use in aromatherapy, as the bark essential oil may cause severe irritation in some people. |
| **Background:** | Cinnamon is one of the oldest spices known. The Chinese and Indians were aware of its medicinal properties over 4,000 years ago. It was also traded with the Egyptians, Greeks and Romans. The British East India Company maintained control of cinnamon production when Sri Lanka was a colony of Britain during the late eighteenth century. |
| **Properties:** | Warming, tonic, stomachic, antispasmodic, |

antiseptic, antifungal, stimulant and haemostatic (stops bleeding).

**Precaution:** This oil is best used in lower concentrations as it may cause irritation in sensitive people.

**Uses:** DIGESTIVE SYSTEM – Warms the stomach and encourages slow digestion when the stomach is cold. Cinnamon can also help flatulence that comes on as a result of eating cold foods.
RESPIRATORY SYSTEM – Valuable for colds and flu, when there are chills and shivering.
REPRODUCTIVE SYSTEM – Good for thrush.
MUSCULAR SYSTEM – Relieves tiredness, cramps and rheumatic and muscular pains.
EMOTION – For mental fatigue and lack of concentration. Cinnamon stimulates and refreshes the mind and eases tension while diminishing the harshness of life. It stimulates the senses and steadies the nerves.

## Blends:

**DIGESTIVE:**
cinnamon 6
ginger 3
orange 3

**RESPIRATORY:**
cinnamon 6
basil 4
benzoin 2

**REPRODUCTIVE:**
cinnamon 4
myrrh 3
lavender 2

**MUSCULAR:**
cinnamon 5
marjoram 4
chamomile (R) 3

**EMOTION:**
cinnamon 5
lemon 3
basil 2

# Citronella

◆ ◇ ◆ ◇ ◆ ◇ ◆ ◇ ◆ ◇ ◆ ◇ ◆ ◇ ◆ ◇ ◆ ◇ ◆ ◇ ◆ ◇ ◆ ◇ ◆ ◇ ◆ ◇ ◆ ◇ ◆ ◇ ◆ ◇ ◆ ◇

| | |
|---|---|
| **Botanical Name:** | *Cymbopogon nardus* |
| **Family:** | *Graminae* |
| **Location:** | It is grown mainly in India, Java and Sri Lanka. |
| **Extraction:** | Steam distillation of the dried leaves. |
| **Colour and Odour:** | The essential oil is pale yellow in colour, having a fresh, lemony and sweet odour. |
| **Description:** | A hardy grass growing to about 90 cm with long slender leaves; it flowers periodically. |
| **Background:** | Introduced into Europe during the nineteenth century. Known universally for its insect-repellent properties. It is used in Europe as a room disinfectant and an air-freshener. Kept in linen cupboards it will keep clothes fresh and deter moths and insects. Citronella is disliked by cats and rodents. |
| **Properties:** | Tonic, stimulant, antiseptic, insecticide and antidepressant. |
| **Precaution:** | This oil is best used in lower concentrations as it may cause irritation in sensitive people. |

**Uses:**  RESPIRATORY SYSTEM – Good for hayfever.
SKIN – It is a deodorant and refreshes sweaty and tired feet. Citronella can be helpful for treating fungal infections.

EMOTION – Eases feelings of depression by its clearing and uplifting effect.

## Blends:

| RESPIRATORY: | | SKIN: | | EMOTION: | |
|---|---|---|---|---|---|
| citronella | 5 | citronella | 5 | citronella | 5 |
| pine | 3 | cypress | 4 | bergamot | 4 |
| eucalyptus | 2 | tea tree | 3 | palmarosa | 2 |

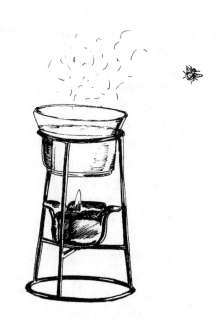

# Clary Sage

| | |
|---|---|
| **Botanical Name:** | *Salvia sclarea* |
| **Family:** | *Labiatae* |
| **Location:** | Clary sage grows in dry soil around the Mediterranean region. Widely cultivated in Russia. |
| **Extraction:** | Steam distillation of the leaves. |
| **Colour and Odour:** | The essential oil is pale yellow in colour with a sweet, slightly floral, nutty and musty scent. |
| **Description:** | A hardy herb growing to 60 cm tall with green, broad, wrinkled leaves and long flowered stalks bearing small blue flowers enclosed by pointed bracts which are green and streaked with purple. |
| **Background:** | Clary sage was highly esteemed in Europe during the Middle Ages. It was introduced into Britain in 1562. In Germany it is used for making muscatel wine and also as a substitute for hops in making beer. The mucilage from clary sage seeds has been used to clear the eyes of foreign particles. In Jamaica, clary sage decoction is boiled in coconut to make a remedy for scorpion stings, and the leaves of clary sage and vervain are used in warm aromatic baths. |
| **Properties:** | Tonic, sedative, hypotensive, anti-convulsant and euphoric. |

**Uses:**   CIRCULATORY SYSTEM – Helpful for reducing high blood pressure.

RESPIRATORY SYSTEM – Relaxes spasms in asthma due to anxiety or other emotional tension.

REPRODUCTIVE SYSTEM – Very useful for treating PMS and period pains. Can also be beneficial for infertility.

NERVOUS SYSTEM – Clary sage's euphoric quality is very good for treating nervous disorders including depression (nervous and post-natal), fearfulness, panic, paranoia and hysteria. Also useful for general debility, and in convalescence.

MUSCULAR SYSTEM – Powerfully relaxant, useful for muscular tension especially when due to mental or emotional stress.

EMOTION – The forceful, profoundly heady and euphoric quality of clary sage is seductive and warm, calming paranoia and stimulating sexuality. Clary sage encourages vivid dreams and dream recall.

## Blends:

**CIRCULATORY:**

| | |
|---|---|
| clary sage | 6 |
| lavender | 3 |
| melissa | 2 |

**RESPIRATORY:**

| | |
|---|---|
| clary sage | 4 |
| benzoin | 3 |
| sandalwood | 3 |

**REPRODUCTIVE:**

| | |
|---|---|
| clary sage | 6 |
| geranium | 3 |
| marjoram | 2 |

**NERVOUS:**

| | |
|---|---|
| clary sage | 5 |
| rose | 3 |
| frankincense | 3 |

**MUSCULAR:**

| | |
|---|---|
| clary sage | 5 |
| rosemary | 4 |
| coriander | 4 |

**EMOTION:**

| | |
|---|---|
| clary sage | 5 |
| ylang-ylang | 4 |
| cedarwood | 3 |

# Clove

◆◇◆◇◆◇◆◇◆◇◆◇◆◇◆◇◆◇◆◇◆◇◆◇◆◇◆◇◆◇◆◇◆◇

| | |
|---|---|
| **Botanical Name:** | *Eugenia caryophyllata* |
| **Family:** | *Myrtaceae* |
| **Location:** | Clove is cultivated in Indonesia. |
| **Extraction:** | Steam distillation of the leaves. |
| **Colour and Odour:** | The essential oil is amber in colour and has a strong, hot, spicy and penetrating aroma. |
| **Description:** | An evergreen tropical tree growing up to 9 m. The flower buds are collected before they open, for distillation. |
| **Background:** | The cultivation of clove was controlled by the Portuguese until the seventeenth century, when it was taken over by the Dutch. Later the French introduced clove trees to their other colonies including Zanzibar, Reunion, Madagascar and a few islands in the Caribbean. Clove is well known as an excellent remedy for soothing toothache and for tooth and gum infections where a strong antiseptic action is required. It is also traditional to use oranges studded with cloves as insect repellents. |
| **Properties:** | Antiseptic, analgesic, carminative, anti-emetic, antispasmodic, antineuralgic and stomachic. |
| **Precaution:** | This oil is best used in lower concentrations as it may cause irritation in sensitive people. |

Uses:   RESPIRATORY SYSTEM – A powerful antiseptic,
useful for colds and flu. Clove is an especially good
preventive during the winter months. It is a good
expectorant, helping to clear mucus and blocked
sinuses. Also helpful for coughs and bronchitis.
REPRODUCTIVE SYSTEM – Tonic and strengthening
in cases of mild impotence.
EMOTION – For mental fatigue, anxiety states and
lack of concentration due to emotional clutter. It
also encourages the mind to recall long-forgotten
memories.

## Blends:

| RESPIRATORY: | | REPRODUCTIVE: | | EMOTION: | |
|---|---|---|---|---|---|
| clove | 4 | clove | 4 | clove | 4 |
| benzoin | 3 | rose | 4 | orange | 4 |
| pine | 3 | lavender | 3 | sandalwood | 4 |

# Coriander

◆ ◇ ◆ ◇ ◆ ◇ ◆ ◇ ◆ ◇ ◆ ◇ ◆ ◇ ◆ ◇ ◆ ◇ ◆ ◇ ◆ ◇ ◆ ◇ ◆ ◇ ◆ ◇ ◆ ◇ ◆ ◇ ◆ ◇ ◆ ◇ ◆ ◇

**Botanical Name:**   *Coriandrum sativum*
**Family:**   *Umbelliferae*
**Location:**   Coriander is cultivated in the Balkan States, Morocco, Rumania and Russia.
**Extraction:**   Steam distillation of the seeds.
**Colour and Odour:**   The essential oil is colourless and has a sweet, spicy-woody aroma.
**Description:**   A small herb growing to 60 cm with bright green, delicate leaves and whitish-pink flowers.
**Background:**   Known to the ancient Egyptians and Greeks, who called it 'koris'(which means 'bug'), as the fresh leaves smell of a squashed bug when crushed. Both the plant and essential oil improve in odour when allowed to age. Coriander is also used in Indian curries.
**Properties:**   Stimulant, carminative, stomachic, anti-spasmodic, antirheumatic and tonic.

**Uses:**   DIGESTIVE SYSTEM – Good for chronic digestive disturbances and a lack of vitality. Stimulates appetite and can be useful for anorexia.
MUSCULAR SYSTEM – Useful for muscular aches and tiredness.
EMOTION – Coriander's warm, provocative scent gently encourages the tired mind into action. Good for mental fatigue and can help with memory.

**Blends:**

| DIGESTIVE: | | MUSCULAR: | | EMOTION: | |
|---|---|---|---|---|---|
| coriander | 7 | coriander | 7 | coriander | 6 |
| lavender | 3 | rosemary | 4 | palmarosa | 3 |
| ginger | 3 | B pepper | 2 | bergamot | 3 |

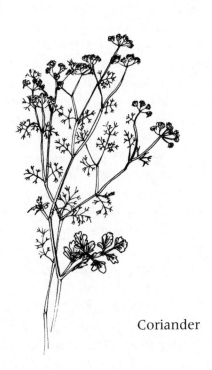

Coriander

# Cumin

◆ ◇ ◆ ◇ ◆ ◇ ◆ ◇ ◆ ◇ ◆ ◇ ◆ ◇ ◆ ◇ ◆ ◇ ◆ ◇ ◆ ◇ ◆ ◇ ◆ ◇ ◆ ◇ ◆ ◇ ◆ ◇ ◆ ◇ ◆ ◇ ◆ ◇

| | |
|---|---|
| **Botanical Name:** | *Cuminum cymimum* |
| **Family:** | *Umbelliferae* |
| **Location:** | Cumin is cultivated in Egypt, India, Morocco and Russia. |
| **Extraction:** | Steam distillation of the seeds. |
| **Colour and Odour:** | The essential oil of cumin is yellow in colour and has a spicy, penetrating and extremely pungent odour. |
| **Description:** | A herb growing up to 30 cm with deep green, fine, thread-like leaves and small white or pink flowers. |
| **Background:** | Used by the Egyptians and the Hebrews since antiquity. It was also highly esteemed by the Greeks and Romans. Introduced to Britain during the Middle Ages. A traditional spice in the Middle East, cumin is nowadays used as an ingredient for Indian curries. |
| **Properties:** | Digestive stimulant, tonic, carminative, antispasmodic, aperitif, emmenagogic and possibly aphrodisiac. |
| **Precaution:** | This oil is best used in lower concentrations as it may cause irritation in sensitive people. The overpowering and lingering odour may be too strong for some individuals. |

**Uses:** DIGESTIVE SYSTEM – Cumin is helpful for sluggish digestion. It relieves griping pains, dyspepsia, flatulence, bloating or diarrhoea.

CIRCULATORY SYSTEM – General tonic and stimulant action on the heart which helps to regulate the metabolic process and is a good remedy for a weak heart and slow circulation.

REPRODUCTIVE SYSTEM – Aphrodisiac action promotes fertility and libido in both men and women. Regulates the menstrual cycle.

MUSCULAR SYSTEM – Warming effect helpful for muscular pains.

SKELETAL SYSTEM – Beneficial for joint pains.

EMOTION – Cumin's strong tonic action on the nervous system helps with tiredness and lethargy. It is powerfully stimulating and penetrates the senses, having an evocative and erotic effect. The odour of cumin induces a sense of protection against negative feelings in oneself and one's environment. Given its unique aroma, it makes a somewhat bizarre, though effective, aphrodisiac.

## Blends:

| DIGESTIVE: | | CIRCULATORY: | | REPRODUCTIVE: | |
|---|---|---|---|---|---|
| cumin | 4 | cumin | 4 | cumin | 4 |
| orange | 4 | rosemary | 4 | neroli | 4 |
| ginger | 4 | melissa | 2 | geranium | 2 |

| MUSCULAR: | | SKELETAL: | | EMOTION: | |
|---|---|---|---|---|---|
| cumin | 4 | cumin | 4 | cumin | 4 |
| coriander | 4 | celery | 4 | mandarin | 4 |
| lavender | 4 | eucalyptus | 4 | ylang-ylang | 4 |

# Cypress

◆◇◆◇◆◇◆◇◆◇◆◇◆◇◆◇◆◇◆◇◆◇◆◇◆◇◆◇◆◇◆◇◆◇

| | |
|---|---|
| **Botanical Name:** | *Cupressus sempervirens* |
| **Family:** | *Cupressaceae* |
| **Location:** | Cypress is found throughout the Mediterranean and is now grown in the Balkan States, France, Italy, North Africa, Portugal and Spain. |
| **Extraction:** | Steam distillation of the cones, leaves or twigs. |
| **Colour and Odour:** | The essential oil is clear with a hint of yellow. It has a woody, nutty and pleasantly smoky aroma with a slightly spicy, resinous undertone. |
| **Description:** | The cypress is a tall, statuesque, conical-shaped evergreen tree. It has a hard, durable wood of a reddish-yellow colour. Furniture made from cypress wood is impervious to insect attacks. |
| **Background:** | Symbolized 'everlastingness' to the ancient Greeks and Romans, who used the wood for building their houses and furniture. The Phoenicians and Cretans also used the wood for building ships. The Egyptians used it for their coffins. The trees are commonly found in churchyards and cemeteries throughout Europe. |
| **Properties:** | Astringent, styptic, antispasmodic, sedative and deodorant. |

Uses: RESPIRATORY SYSTEM – Very useful for all respiratory problems with spasms, such as whooping cough and asthma. Also useful for influenza, bronchitis and emphysema.

CIRCULATORY SYSTEM – Beneficial for heavy periods. It has a vaso-constricting effect, good for haemorrhoids and varicose veins.

REPRODUCTIVE SYSTEM – Valuable in the treatment of menopausal symptoms such as hot flushes and irritability, and menstrual problems such as premenstrual tension.

SKIN – Good for excessive perspiration and for deodorizing sweaty feet.

EMOTION – Cypress is soothing in times of transition, whether moving home or changing career, when the changes are difficult or painful. It is particularly strengthening and comforting when ending relationships or during bereavement. It eases the sadness and helps to strengthen the bereaved. Cypress is an ancient symbol of solace. Also good for sluggish minds.

## Blends:

**RESPIRATORY:**

| | |
|---|---|
| cypress | 7 |
| benzoin | 3 |
| frankincense | 3 |

**CIRCULATORY:**

| | |
|---|---|
| cypress | 7 |
| chamomile (G) | 4 |
| geranium | 2 |

**REPRODUCTIVE:**

| | |
|---|---|
| cypress | 7 |
| clary sage | 3 |
| geranium | 2 |

**SKIN:**

| | |
|---|---|
| cypress | 7 |
| tea tree | 4 |
| peppermint | 2 |

**EMOTION:**

| | |
|---|---|
| cypress | 6 |
| rose | 4 |
| frankincense | 2 |

# Eucalyptus

| | |
|---|---|
| **Botanical Name:** | *Eucalyptus globulus* |
| **Family:** | *Myrtaceae* |
| **Location:** | The eucalyptus tree is indigenous to Australia. It is now cultivated in many sub-tropical regions including Algeria, southern China, Egypt, India, South Africa, Spain, and also in the state of California. |
| **Extraction:** | Steam distillation of the leaves. |
| **Colour and Odour:** | The essential oil is colourless and has a distinct, crisp, camphoraceous odour that is penetrating and refreshing. |
| **Description:** | Some species of eucalyptus grow up to 135 m and are among the tallest trees in the world. The trees are also deeply rooted and grow incredibly fast, forming a fairly strong wood that is resistant to rot. Some species of eucalyptus yield a gum. |
| **Background:** | It was introduced to Europe and the rest of the world from Australia in 1857. The trees are usually planted in swampy areas to prevent the spread of malaria. However, when grown outside Australia it tends to secrete substances that inhibit the growth of surrounding plants. |
| **Properties:** | Antiseptic, expectorant, slightly antispasmodic, mildly astringent, analgesic, rubefacient, bactericidal and antiviral. |

**Uses:** RESPIRATORY SYSTEM – An extremely effective remedy for reducing body temperature in all types of fever. Valuable as a decongestant for catarrh in most respiratory tract infections including colds, influenza, sinusitis, tuberculosis and throat infections, especially when there is a purulent mucus discharge. Provides good protection during epidemics. Eucalyptus is useful for hay fever.

NERVOUS SYSTEM – Analgesic in neuralgia and congestive headaches.

MUSCULAR SYSTEM – Good for general muscular aches and pains.

SKELETAL SYSTEM – Beneficial for rheumatoid arthritis and helps to remove toxins in the joints.

SKIN – Good for skin eruptions, shingles, herpes, indolent wounds, ulcers and burns.

EMOTION – Clears the head of mental exhaustion and the inability to concentrate. Balances extremes of mood. Eucalyptus cools heated emotions when people are engaged in any form of combat, be it verbal, emotional or physical. Its aroma creates a feeling of space.

## Blends:

**RESPIRATORY:**
eucalyptus 7
pine 3
benzoin 3

**NERVOUS:**
eucalyptus 7
lavender 4
peppermint 2

**MUSCULAR:**
eucalyptus 6
chamomile (R) 5
lavender 3

**SKELETAL:**
eucalyptus 7
juniper 4
rosemary 3

**SKIN:**
eucalyptus 5
lavender 4
tea tree 3

**EMOTION:**
eucalyptus 5
lemon 4
basil 3

# Fennel

◆ ◇ ◆ ◇ ◆ ◇ ◆ ◇ ◆ ◇ ◆ ◇ ◆ ◇ ◆ ◇ ◆ ◇ ◆ ◇ ◆ ◇ ◆ ◇ ◆ ◇ ◆ ◇ ◆ ◇ ◆ ◇

| | |
|---|---|
| **Botanical Name:** | *Foeniculum vulgare* |
| **Family:** | *Umbelliferae* |
| **Location:** | Fennel is found all over the Mediterranean region and it is cultivated in Bulgaria, France, Germany, Hungary, Italy, Portugal, Spain and North Africa. |
| **Extraction:** | Steam distillation of the seeds. |
| **Colour and Odour:** | The essential oil is colourless and has a very sweet and somewhat warm, anisic aroma. |
| **Description:** | A herb growing up to 1.2 m with bright green, feathery leaves and golden yellow flowers. Found mainly on limestone soil, especially near the sea. |
| **Background:** | Known to the early Greeks and Romans and grown in Europe as a popular vegetable often eaten with fish. Fennel is one of the main constituents of babies' gripe water. |
| **Properties:** | Carminative, diuretic, stimulant, antispasmodic, anti-inflammatory and tonic. |

**Uses:**   DIGESTIVE SYSTEM – An excellent carminative and digestive remedy for indigestion and flatulence. Tones the muscles of the digestive tract. Counteracts the effects of alcohol consumption; useful for recovering alcoholics.

102

URINARY SYSTEM – Fennel's cleansing action clears toxins from the body. Its diuretic action promotes the flow of urine and helps with water retention and obesity.

REPRODUCTIVE SYSTEM – Helps to regulate menstruation when periods are scanty and painful. Valuable for treating menopausal problems. Also promotes milk flow.

SKELETAL SYSTEM – Helpful for gouty conditions.

SKIN – Valuable for treating cellulite by helping to detoxify the accumulation of wastes.

EMOTION – Fennel energizes, comforts and enlivens the mind. It induces a sense of courage, caution and calmness.

## Blends:

| DIGESTIVE: | | URINARY: | | REPRODUCTIVE: | |
|---|---|---|---|---|---|
| fennel | 6 | fennel | 6 | fennel | 5 |
| orange | 4 | juniper | 4 | cypress | 4 |
| peppermint | 2 | rosemary | 3 | clary sage | 3 |

| SKELETAL: | | SKIN: | | EMOTION: | |
|---|---|---|---|---|---|
| fennel | 6 | fennel | 5 | fennel | 5 |
| lemon | 4 | celery | 4 | lemon | 4 |
| chamomile (G) | 2 | juniper | 4 | juniper | 3 |

# Frankincense

**Botanical Name:** *Boswellia carterii*
**Family:** *Burseraceae*
**Location:** Frankincense grows wild in the deserts of Somalia, Ethiopia and Saudi Arabia.
**Extraction:** Steam distillation of the gum-resin.
**Colour and Odour:** The essential oil is colourless with a warm, balsamic, spicy aroma that is dry and fortifying with sweet undertones.
**Description:** A small tree, it has small leaves and pale pink flowers. The whole tree has abundant resin that exudes a milky juice which hardens to 'tears' on exposure to the air. The solid 'tears' are then collected.
**Background:** Frankincense was among the earliest incenses, with 3,000 years of continual religious usage. Valued as highly as gold, it was long used by the Egyptians for religious and ceremonial purposes. Mentioned several times in the Bible.
**Properties:** Antiseptic, sedative, tonic, cytophylactic, cicatrizant, expectorant, astringent and anti-inflammatory.

**Uses:** RESPIRATORY SYSTEM – Slows down and deepens the breathing, ensuring calm and comfort. Very useful for asthma, particularly for those sufferers with a fearful disposition.

SKIN – Rejuvenating for the skin; especially good for ageing skin and wrinkles, and for preserving a youthful complexion. Effective for healing wounds, scars and injuries.

EMOTION – Reduces tension. Frankincense calms the physical form and awakens the higher consciousness. It produces a heightened awareness of the spiritual realm and deepens religious experience. Frankincense is ideal for use prior to meditation. Offers strength in the face of adversity and hardship, and protection from the material world, bringing enlightenment, releasing subconscious stress and lifting the spirits.

## Blends:

| RESPIRATORY: | | SKIN: | | EMOTION: | |
|---|---|---|---|---|---|
| frankincense | 7 | frankincense | 4 | frankincense | 7 |
| benzoin | 3 | rose | 3 | cedarwood | 3 |
| lavender | 2 | neroli | 2 | mandarin | 2 |

# Geranium

◆ ◇ ◆ ◇ ◆ ◇ ◆ ◇ ◆ ◇ ◆ ◇ ◆ ◇ ◆ ◇ ◆ ◇ ◆ ◇ ◆ ◇ ◆ ◇ ◆ ◇ ◆ ◇ ◆ ◇ ◆ ◇

| | |
|---|---|
| **Botanical Name:** | *Pelargonium graveolens* |
| **Family:** | *Geraniaceae* |
| **Location:** | Geranium is cultivated in China, Egypt and Reunion. |
| **Extraction:** | Steam distillation of the leaves. |
| **Colour and Odour:** | The essential oil is light green in colour and has a delightfully fresh, sweet and heavy rose-like aroma. |
| **Description:** | A shrub of about 60 cm high with serrated, pointed leaves and small pink flowers. Much cultivated in window boxes and tubs. It is an easy plant to grow in a warm climate. In cooler climates it does well indoors. |
| **Background:** | Geranium is related to the cranesbill, valued as a medicinal herb. Native to South Africa, commercial production of geranium oil began in the early nineteenth century by the French, but nowadays the major production region is in the former French colony of Bourbon, now called Reunion, an island in the southwest Indian Ocean. |
| **Properties:** | Tonic, astringent, mildly analgesic, sedative, anti-inflammatory, nervine, calming and antispasmodic. |

**Uses:**    URINARY SYSTEM – Tonic effect on the kidneys and a mild diuretic, of value in treating urinary tract infections.

ENDOCRINE SYSTEM – Geranium balances the secretion of hormones and stimulates the lymphatic system and the pancreas.

REPRODUCTIVE SYSTEM – Very useful in treating menopausal problems such as hot flushes and night sweats and to relieve premenstrual tension. Its draining qualities are useful for engorgement of the breasts.

SKIN – Geranium is a mild skin tonic. It is a cleansing and refreshing astringent, useful for all skin conditions and for almost any skin type. It balances the production of sebum and is therefore good for both excessively dry skin or congested, oily skin. A valuable aid in the treatment of cellulite. Geranium is good for all types of wounds.

EMOTION – Geranium is both calming and refreshing to the psyche at the same time. It is successful in lifting depression and treating anxiety states. It balances the mind and helps us to gain control of our lives again when we are feeling depleted and blue. A mood adjuster.

## Blends:

**URINARY:**
| | |
|---|---|
| geranium | 6 |
| juniper | 4 |
| rosemary | 3 |

**ENDOCRINE:**
| | |
|---|---|
| geranium | 6 |
| sandalwood | 3 |
| clary sage | 3 |

**REPRODUCTIVE:**
| | |
|---|---|
| geranium | 6 |
| neroli | 3 |
| lavender | 2 |

**SKIN:**
| | |
|---|---|
| geranium | 4 |
| rose | 3 |
| bergamot | 2 |

**EMOTION:**
| | |
|---|---|
| geranium | 5 |
| grapefruit | 4 |
| ylang-ylang | 2 |

# Ginger

◆ ◇ ◆ ◇ ◆ ◇ ◆ ◇ ◆ ◇ ◆ ◇ ◆ ◇ ◆ ◇ ◆ ◇ ◆ ◇ ◆ ◇ ◆ ◇ ◆ ◇ ◆ ◇ ◆ ◇ ◆ ◇

| | |
|---|---|
| **Botanical Name:** | *Zingiber officinale* |
| **Family:** | *Zingiberaceae* |
| **Location:** | Ginger is native to tropical Asia. It is extensively cultivated in China, Guatemala, India, Jamaica, Japan and Nigeria. |
| **Extraction:** | Steam distillation of the rhizome (roots). |
| **Colour and Odour:** | The essential oil is yellow in colour with a warm, fresh, spicy aroma. |
| **Description:** | A perennial herb with an erect, reed-like, white-flowering stem rising from a creeping, jointed rhizome. |
| **Background:** | Used by the Chinese and Indians for its medicinal properties for thousands of years. Known to the ancient Greeks and Romans. Introduced to Europe by the Arabs between the 10th and 15th centuries; later introduced into South America by the Spaniards. |
| **Properties:** | Warming, aperitif, carminative, stimulant, stomachic and tonic. |
| **Precaution:** | This oil should not be used when there is excessive heat or inflammation, and is best used in lower concentrations as it may cause irritation in sensitive people. |

**Uses:**     DIGESTIVE SYSTEM – Has a warming action on the stomach and slows digestion.

RESPIRATORY SYSTEM – Ginger is powerfully expectorant, clearing the lungs of accumulated catarrh and mucus. Also good for congested sinuses or colds, flu and bronchitis, especially with chills or shivering. Beneficial to bronchial asthma.

NERVOUS SYSTEM – Helpful for travel sickness and 'morning sickness' in pregnancy, reducing nausea and vomiting.

MUSCULAR SYSTEM – Massaged into the limbs, ginger increases the flow of blood to the extremities for cold, rheumatic pains in the hands and feet.

SKELETAL SYSTEM – Very helpful for warming swollen joints aggravated by external dampness.

EMOTION – Warms the emotions, sharpens the senses, aids the memory and is grounding.

## Blends:

**DIGESTIVE:**

| | |
|---|---|
| ginger | 5 |
| cardamon | 3 |
| fennel | 3 |

**RESPIRATORY:**

| | |
|---|---|
| ginger | 6 |
| benzoin | 3 |
| frankincense | 3 |

**NERVOUS:**

| | |
|---|---|
| ginger | 4 |
| lavender | 2 |
| peppermint | 2 |

**MUSCULAR:**

| | |
|---|---|
| ginger | 6 |
| coriander | 4 |
| rosemary | 3 |

**SKELETAL:**

| | |
|---|---|
| ginger | 6 |
| chamomile (R) | 3 |
| camphor | 2 |

**EMOTION:**

| | |
|---|---|
| ginger | 5 |
| mandarin | 4 |
| orange | 3 |

# Grapefruit

◆ ◇ ◆ ◇ ◆ ◇ ◆ ◇ ◆ ◇ ◆ ◇ ◆ ◇ ◆ ◇ ◆ ◇ ◆ ◇ ◆ ◇ ◆ ◇ ◆ ◇ ◆ ◇ ◆ ◇ ◆ ◇ ◆ ◇

**Botanical Name:** *Citrus paradisi*

**Family:** *Rutaceae*

**Location:** Grapefruit is extensively cultivated in Brazil, California and Florida.

**Extraction:** Expression of the peel.

**Colour and Odour:** The essential oil is yellow in colour with a light, fresh, tangy, sweet aroma.

**Description:** An evergreen tree with shiny leaves, white flowers and large yellow fruits, which are much larger than oranges.

**Background:** Grapefruit is widely used as a breakfast fruit and also for its juice. The essential oil is used in perfumery, especially toilet water.

**Properties:** Antidepressant, antiseptic, diuretic, stimulant and tonic.

**Uses:** DIGESTIVE SYSTEM – Stimulates the appetite, acts as a tonic to the stomach and liver and promotes digestive secretions.

URINARY SYSTEM – Promotes kidney function by helping to eliminate water, therefore useful for obesity and water retention. Also has a cleansing effect on the kidneys, helping to eliminate toxins from the body.

EMOTION – Grapefruit has a balancing effect on the emotions. It is uplifting, brightening up dark, depressive moods and boosting confidence. It helps

110

with procrastination, frustration and bitterness.
May even help to stabilize manic depression.

**Blends:**

| DIGESTIVE: | | URINARY: | | EMOTION: | |
|---|---|---|---|---|---|
| grapefruit | 7 | grapefruit | 7 | grapefruit | 7 |
| coriander | 3 | juniper | 3 | sandalwood | 3 |
| carrot | 2 | fennel | 2 | lavender | 2 |

# Hyssop

| | |
|---|---|
| **Botanical Name:** | *Hyssopus officinalis* |
| **Family:** | *Labiatae* |
| **Location:** | Hyssop grows wild throughout the Mediterranean region and is cultivated in Albania, the Balkan States, France and Hungary. |
| **Extraction:** | Steam distillation of the leaves. |
| **Colour and Odour:** | The essential oil is pale yellow in colour and has a deep, penetrating, warm aroma with sweet undertones. |
| **Description:** | A small herb growing up to 60 cm in height with slim, pointed leaves and pale blue flowers. It grows in warm, dry, hilly places, especially on rocky slopes and sunny meadows. |
| **Background:** | Long known for its cleansing properties by the Greeks and Romans. Popular with the Benedictine monks during the tenth century, it is one of the main ingredients of Chartreuse liqueur. |
| **Properties:** | Stimulating, tonic, sedative, expectorant, hypertensive, antiseptic and antispasmodic. |
| **Precaution:** | This oil is best used in lower concentrations as it may cause irritation in sensitive people. |

Uses:   CIRCULATORY SYSTEM – An excellent regulator of
blood pressure and a fine tonic in states of
weakness and during convalescence. It is beneficial
for cardiovascular disorders.
RESPIRATORY SYSTEM – Valuable in respiratory
disorders as it liquefies mucus, promotes
expectoration and relieves bronchial spasms. An
excellent cough remedy. Beneficial for all catarrhal
conditions, influenza and bronchitis.
NERVOUS SYSTEM – A nerve sedative and tonic,
hyssop strengthens the nerves and aids relaxation.
SKIN – Very good for bruises and wounds.
EMOTION – Clears the mind, giving a feeling of
alertness. Brings deep emotions into focus,
producing clarity.

## Blends:

| CIRCULATORY: | | RESPIRATORY: | | NERVOUS: | |
|---|---|---|---|---|---|
| hyssop | 4 | hyssop | 4 | hyssop | 4 |
| ylang-ylang | 3 | sandalwood | 3 | jasmine | 4 |
| rose | 3 | cajeput | 3 | lavender | 2 |

| SKIN: | | EMOTION: | |
|---|---|---|---|
| hyssop | 4 | hyssop | 4 |
| myrrh | 4 | lemon | 4 |
| cypress | 2 | ylang-ylang | 3 |

# Jasmine

◆ ◇ ◆ ◇ ◆ ◇ ◆ ◇ ◆ ◇ ◆ ◇ ◆ ◇ ◇ ◆ ◇ ◆ ◇ ◆ ◇ ◆ ◇ ◆ ◇ ◆ ◇ ◆ ◇ ◆ ◇ ◆ ◇

| | |
|---|---|
| **Botanical Name:** | *Jasminum grandiflorum* |
| **Family:** | *Oleaceae* |
| **Location:** | Jasmine is native to China and India; it is cultivated in Egypt, France, Italy, Morocco and Turkey. |
| **Extraction:** | Solvent extraction of the flowers. |
| **Colour and Odour:** | The absolute is a deep reddish-brown in colour and has a warm, sweet, exotic, slightly heady aroma with a hint of musky undertones. |
| **Description:** | A creeping vine with dark green leaves and delicate white flowers growing up to 6 m in height. |
| **Background:** | Long used in China as a perfume and for scenting tea. It is fashionable for Chinese girls to wear jasmine flowers in their hair. Jasmine is also important in the Hindu and Muslim traditions, and was introduced by the Moors to Spain. Used in Malaya for fevers. Jasmine is now one of the most expensive perfume ingredients. |
| **Properties:** | Sedative, uplifting, antidepressant, anti-spasmodic and aphrodisiac. |

**Uses:**     REPRODUCTIVE SYSTEM – Relieves uterine spasms and menstrual cramps. Very useful during child birth.

SKIN – Good for dry, sensitive skin, especially

when there is redness. Jasmine also increases skin
elasticity.
EMOTION – Dispels apathy, indifference and listlessness,
producing feelings of optimism, confidence and
euphoria. It releases inhibitions, liberates imagination
and is exhilarating. Jasmine powerfully provokes
fantasies, lifting the darkest moods and bringing out
inner desires. It is beneficial for postnatal depression.
Jasmine is a known aphrodisiac.

## Blends:

| REPRODUCTIVE: | | SKIN: | | EMOTION: | |
|---|---|---|---|---|---|
| jasmine | 5 | jasmine | 3 | jasmine | 4 |
| geranium | 3 | lavender | 2 | mandarin | 4 |
| marjoram | 2 | chamomile (R) | 2 | sandalwood | 3 |

# Juniper

◆◇◆◇◆◇◆◇◆◇◆◇◆◇◆◇◆◇◆◇◆◇◆◇◆◇◆◇◆◇◆◇◆◇

**Botanical Name:** *Juniperus communis*

**Family:** *Cupressaceae*

**Location:** Juniper is found in North America, northern Europe, and from Siberia to southwest Asia.

**Extraction:** Steam distillation of the deep-blue ripe berries.

**Colour and Odour:** The essential oil is colourless and has a fresh, pleasing aroma.

**Description:** The juniper tree is a small evergreen growing to about 9 m with short spiny leaves and berries which are blue-black in colour. The berries take about two years to ripen. It is commonly found all over Europe in chalky or lime soils.

**Background:** Known by the ancient Egyptians and Greeks and used to combat epidemics. Around the time of the First World War, French hospitals used juniper in the sick wards as incense to combat diseases such as smallpox. Juniper berries are used in making gin.

**Properties:** Antiseptic, antirheumatic, depurative, diuretic, detoxifying, emmenagogic, purifying, rubefacient, stimulant and tonic.

Uses:       DIGESTIVE SYSTEM – Useful for indigestion, minor
            stomach upsets, flatulence and colic.
            URINARY SYSTEM – Juniper is a strong antiseptic
            and diuretic for treating cystitis and kidney
            inflammation. Good for alleviating water
            retention.
            RESPIRATORY SYSTEM – A respiratory tract
            antiseptic, juniper is also good for convulsive
            coughs.
            SKELETAL SYSTEM – Arthritic and joint problems,
            such as gout, will benefit from juniper.
            SKIN – Good for disorders of the skin. Cleansing
            and toning, juniper is especially useful for treating
            oily skin and acne. Detoxifying for cellulite.
            EMOTION – Useful for treating sleep difficulties due
            to worry and tension. Juniper strengthens anyone
            feeling emotionally drained. It is particularly
            good for cleansing the mind of negative vibes
            accumulated from others. It revitalizes people who
            are cold and aloof and feel as though they are
            misunderstood and unsupported.

**Blends:**

| DIGESTIVE: | | URINARY: | | RESPIRATORY: | |
|---|---|---|---|---|---|
| juniper | 7 | juniper | 6 | juniper | 6 |
| parsley | 3 | celery | 4 | eucalyptus | 3 |
| fennel | 2 | sandalwood | 2 | sandalwood | 3 |

| SKELETAL: | | SKIN: | | EMOTION: | |
|---|---|---|---|---|---|
| juniper | 7 | juniper | 6 | juniper | 6 |
| eucalyptus | 4 | rosemary | 3 | bergamot | 4 |
| chamomile (G) | 3 | chamomile (R) | 3 | frankincense | 2 |

117

# Lavender

◆◇◆◇◆◇◆◇◆◇◆◇◆◇◆◇◆◇◆◇◆◇◆◇◆◇◆◇◆◇◆◇

| | |
|---|---|
| **Botanical Name:** | *Lavendula officinalis* |
| **Family:** | *Labiatae* |
| **Location:** | Lavender grows wild along the Mediterranean coast but is also extensively cultivated for its fragrance in England and France. |
| **Extraction:** | Steam distillation of the flowers. |
| **Colour and Odour:** | The essential oil is clear with a hint of yellow. It has a fresh, sweet floral scent. |
| **Description:** | A shrub growing to about 90 cm tall having narrow, linear, grey-green leaves and beautiful blue-violet flowers borne on long spikes. |
| **Background:** | Probably introduced by the Romans to England, lavender quickly became popular for strewing, in pot-pourris, and is also widely used in toilet water. Lavender is the most versatile and useful essential oil for therapeutic purposes. |
| **Properties:** | Sedative, tonic, hypotensive, analgesic, antiseptic, antispasmodic, diuretic, cytophylactic and balancing. |
| **For those who wish to cultivate their own lavender:** | Lavender is able to withstand cold winters in Britain, although it is a native of the warm Mediterranean. It can be propogated either by seed or cuttings. If growing from seeds, they must be kept in humid sand to |

bring out germination, after which they should be transplanted into nurseries and watered frequently for several months, when they are finally ready for planting in the open fields. Stem cuttings about 4–8 in long are taken in autumn and spring and planted 18 in apart, deep and very firmly in the soil, in cold frames where they root readily.

Lavender cultivation should be carried out in open and sunny sites to discourage fungus disease. Farmlands of insufficient fertility, abandoned for many years, are particularly suited. In Britain, land with a southern exposure is ideal. Rainy weather may produce a fair crop of flowers but the yield of oil will be very poor. If improperly cultivated and the crop starts to decline in the fifth year, planting should be renewed. English lavender differs from French lavender in odour by being more camphoraceous and less sweet. This is the typical English lavender scent that many have recognized over the generations.

Uses:   URINARY SYSTEM – Beneficial for cystitis.
CIRCULATORY SYSTEM – Valuable in the treatment of palpitations and high blood pressure.
RESPIRATORY SYSTEM – Beneficial for treating throat infections, influenza, bronchitis and whooping cough. Helps asthma sufferers when their condition is associated with mental or emotional trauma.
REPRODUCTIVE SYSTEM – Useful for treating

scanty menstruation and leucorrhoea.

NERVOUS SYSTEM – Calms a variety of nervous disorders including excitability, insomnia, migraine and nervous tension. Lavender is also good for other nervous problems such as panic, hysteria, trembling, convulsion and epilepsy. Particularly good for depression and delusions.

MUSCULAR SYSTEM – Good for muscular and rheumatic aches and pains.

SKELETAL SYSTEM – Beneficial for general joint pains.

SKIN – An excellent skin rejuvenator, good for stretch-marks. It is antiseptic and may be used with benefit on all skin types. Useful for inflammation, dermatitis, eczema, psoriasis, boils, scarring and burns. Lavender is also a very effective remedy for sunburn, insect bites and stings.

EMOTION – A steadying influence on the psyche, removing indecisiveness and emotional conflict. Lavender's balancing effect calms stormy or uncontrolled emotional states by bringing the feelings under conscious control. Tempers extreme emotional states with a sense of rationality. Generally strengthens the conscious mind, emanating a noble, mellow peacefulness. Good for depression.

**Blends:**

URINARY:
lavender 6
sandalwood 4
juniper 2

CIRCULATORY:
lavender 7
ylang-ylang 3
melissa 2

RESPIRATORY:
lavender 6
benzoin 4
cedarwood 2

**REPRODUCTIVE:**

| | |
|---|---|
| lavender | 6 |
| sandalwood | 4 |
| rose | 3 |

**NERVOUS:**

| | |
|---|---|
| lavender | 7 |
| frankincense | 3 |
| rose | 3 |

**MUSCULAR:**

| | |
|---|---|
| lavender | 7 |
| coriander | 3 |
| nutmeg | 3 |

**SKELETAL:**

| | |
|---|---|
| lavender | 7 |
| rosemary | 4 |
| chamomile (G) | 3 |

**SKIN:**

| | |
|---|---|
| lavender | 4 |
| chamomile (R) | 2 |
| sandalwood | 2 |

**EMOTION:**

| | |
|---|---|
| lavender | 6 |
| neroli | 3 |
| petitgrain | 2 |

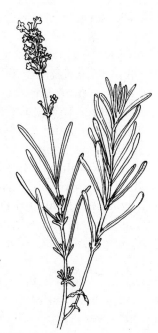

Lavender

# Lemon

| | |
|---|---|
| **Botanical Name:** | *Citrus limonum* |
| **Family:** | *Rutaceae* |
| **Location:** | Lemons are widely grown in tropical America, California, Florida, Israel, Italy and Spain. |
| **Extraction:** | Expression of the peel. |
| **Colour and Odour:** | The essential oil is yellow in colour and has a crisp, clean scent. |
| **Description:** | A thorny evergreen tree growing to about 1.8 m with shiny oval leaves and pinkish-white fragrant flowers, the fruits turning from green to yellow when ripe. |
| **Background:** | Introduced from the East into Europe by the Italians during the fifth century and later also cultivated in Spain and Portugal. The fresh fruit and juice have long been used as food flavourings. |
| **Properties:** | Haemostatic, antibacterial, tonic, hypotensive and sedative. |

**Uses:** DIGESTIVE SYSTEM – Good general tonic to the digestive tract, especially the stomach and liver.
CIRCULATORY SYSTEM – Especially useful for treating high blood pressure, hardening of the arteries and varicose veins.
RESPIRATORY SYSTEM – Of great value in treating bronchitis and influenza.

SKELETAL SYSTEM – Lemon helps to eliminate the toxins which causes arthritic and gouty pain.

SKIN – Lemon helps to stop bleeding in minor cuts and wounds. Good for greasy skin. Brightens pale and dull complexions and may also be helpful for lightening freckles.

EMOTION – The clean, fresh, lively scent dispels sluggishness, indecision and lack of humour, stimulates the body into action and aids clear thinking.

## Blends:

| DIGESTIVE: | | CIRCULATORY: | | RESPIRATORY: | |
|---|---|---|---|---|---|
| lemon | 7 | lemon | 7 | lemon | 6 |
| coriander | 3 | ylang-ylang | 4 | eucalyptus | 3 |
| cardamon | 2 | lavender | 2 | benzoin | 2 |

| SKELETAL: | | SKIN: | | EMOTION: | |
|---|---|---|---|---|---|
| lemon | 7 | lemon | 3 | lemon | 7 |
| juniper | 4 | neroli | 2 | bergamot | 3 |
| chamomile (G) | 3 | lavender | 2 | anise | 2 |

# Lemongrass

◆ ◇ ◆ ◇ ◆ ◇ ◆ ◇ ◆ ◇ ◆ ◇ ◆ ◇ ◆ ◇ ◆ ◇ ◆ ◇ ◆ ◇ ◆ ◇ ◆ ◇ ◆ ◇ ◆ ◇ ◆ ◇ ◆ ◇

| | |
|---|---|
| **Botanical Name:** | *Cymbopogon citratus* |
| **Family:** | *Graminae* |
| **Location:** | Lemongrass is grown in Africa, Guatemala, India and Sri Lanka. |
| **Extraction:** | Steam distillation of the leaves. |
| **Colour and Odour:** | The essential oil is golden-yellow with a strong, sweet, lemony scent. |
| **Description:** | A tropical aromatic grass growing to 90 cm in height in India (slightly taller or shorter when grown elsewhere). |
| **Background:** | Long used in India especially for fevers and infectious diseases. Very useful as a room freshener and deodorizer. |
| **Properties:** | Tonic, stimulant, strong antiseptic, bactericide, refreshing and deodorant. |
| **Precaution:** | This oil is best used in lower concentrations as it may cause irritation in sensitive people. |

**Uses:**   RESPIRATORY SYSTEM – Helpful in preventing respiratory infections, sore throats and laryngitis.
MUSCULAR SYSTEM – Helps to tone muscles and make them more supple.
EMOTION – Lemongrass is purifying and stimulates awareness. It refreshes the mind and is helpful for mental fatigue and loss of concentration.

## Blends:

| RESPIRATORY: | | MUSCULAR: | | EMOTION: | |
|---|---|---|---|---|---|
| lemongrass | 5 | lemongrass | 5 | lemongrass | 4 |
| eucalyptus | 4 | rosemary | 4 | orange | 4 |
| sandalwood | 3 | coriander | 3 | basil | 2 |

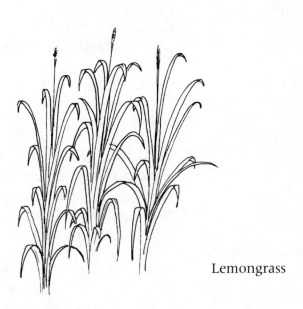

Lemongrass

# Lime

◆ ◇ ◆ ◇ ◆ ◇ ◆ ◇ ◆ ◇ ◆ ◇ ◆ ◇ ◆ ◇ ◆ ◇ ◆ ◇ ◆ ◇ ◆ ◇ ◆ ◇ ◆ ◇ ◆ ◇

| | |
|---|---|
| **Botanical name:** | *Citrus aurantifolia* |
| **Family:** | *Rutaceae* |
| **Location:** | Lime is cultivated in Italy and tropical America. |
| **Extraction:** | Expression of the peel. |
| **Colour and Odour:** | The essential oil is clear with a hint of yellow. It has a fresh, sweet, zesty aroma. |
| **Description:** | A small thorny evergreen tree growing to about 3 m high with smooth oval leaves and small white flowers. The lime resembles the lemon in appearance but is more rounded and greener. The fruits are generally about 5 cm long. |
| **Background:** | The lime tree originated in the East and was introduced to Europe by the Moors and to tropical America by the Portuguese and Spaniards in the sixteenth century. Royal Navy ships used to stock up with limes to prevent scurvy among the sailors, thus British sailors came to be known as 'limeys'. |
| **Properties:** | Antiseptic, astringent, restorative and tonic. |

**Uses:** DIGESTIVE SYSTEM – A digestive stimulant, encouraging appetite. Useful for treating anorexia.
SKIN – Toning and astringent for a greasy skin and scalp. Also good for wounds.

EMOTION – Very refreshing and uplifting to a tired mind; energizing and revitalizing for depression.

## Blends:

| DIGESTIVE: | | SKIN: | | EMOTION: | |
|---|---|---|---|---|---|
| lime | 7 | lime | 5 | lime | 6 |
| B pepper | 3 | lavender | 3 | bergamot | 3 |
| coriander | 2 | mandarin | 2 | rosemary | 2 |

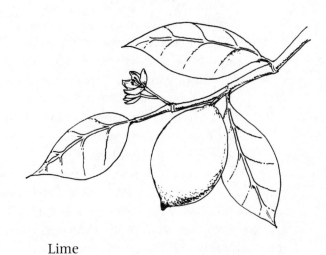

Lime

# Mandarin

◆ ◇ ◆ ◇ ◆ ◇ ◆ ◇ ◆ ◇ ◆ ◇ ◆ ◇ ◆ ◇ ◆ ◇ ◆ ◇ ◆ ◇ ◆ ◇ ◆ ◇ ◆ ◇ ◆ ◇ ◆ ◇ ◆ ◇ ◆ ◇

| | |
|---|---|
| **Botanical Name:** | *Citrus nobilis* |
| **Family:** | *Rutaceae* |
| **Location:** | Mandarin is grown in Algeria, Brazil, California, Cyprus, Florida, Greece, Italy, Spain and Texas. |
| **Extraction:** | Expression of the peel. |
| **Colour and Odour:** | The essential oil is golden yellow in colour and has a delicate, sweet (almost floral) aroma reminiscent of the fruit itself. |
| **Description:** | A small evergreen tree growing up to about 5.4 m with shiny oval leaves, fragrant flowers and fleshy fruits with skins that peel off easily. The mandarin is very similar to the tangerine. The taste and flavour of both are more delicate and refined than those of the orange. |
| **Background:** | Originating in China, where it is traditionally very important, the fruit was named after the Chinese mandarins. It was introduced to Europe at the beginning of the nineteenth century and to the Americas about half a century later. |
| **Properties:** | Antispasmodic, cytophylactic, digestive, sedative and tonic. |

**Uses:**     DIGESTIVE SYSTEM – Aids digestion as it calms the intestines but acts as a tonic for the stomach and liver. Gentle action suitable for treating hiccups.

**SKIN** – Promotes cell regeneration; excellent for pregnancy; prevents stretch marks.

**EMOTION** – Fresh, subtle, sympathetic, inspiring and strengthening.

## Blends:

| DIGESTIVE: | | SKIN: | | EMOTION: | |
|---|---|---|---|---|---|
| mandarin | 6 | mandarin | 6 | mandarin | 7 |
| fennel | 4 | frankincense | 3 | frankincense | 3 |
| coriander | 2 | lavender | 3 | rosewood | 2 |

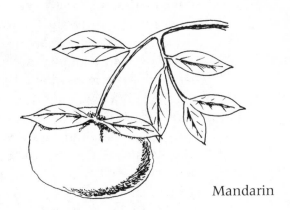

Mandarin

# Marjoram

◆ ◇ ◆ ⌃ ◆ ◡ ◆ ◡ ◆ ◇ ◆ ◡ ◆ ◡ ◆ ◇ ◆ ◇ ◆ ◇ ◆ ◇ ◆ ◇ ◆ ◇ ◆ ◇ ◆ ◇ ◆ ◇ ◆ ◇ ◆ ◇ ◆ ◇

| | |
|---|---|
| Botanical Name: | *Origanum marjorana* |
| Family: | *Labiatae* |
| Location: | Marjoram is grown in Bulgaria, Egypt, Germany, Hungary, Morocco and Tunisia. |
| Extraction: | Steam distillation of the leaves. |
| Colour and Odour: | The essential oil is colourless with a warm, sharp, spicy aroma. |
| Description: | A tender bush growing up to about 30 cm with a hairy stem, small, soft, velvety oval leaves and pinkish-white flowers. It prefers the light, warm soils of gardens. |
| Background: | As well as being a popular herb in cookery, marjoram has a reputation for promoting long life. It is a joyful herb given to newlyweds and planted in graveyards to bring peace. Marjoram was very popular with the ancient Greeks, who used it in their perfumes, cosmetics and medicine. |
| Properties: | Sedative, antispasmodic, hypotensive, analgesic and carminative. |

Uses:    DIGESTIVE SYSTEM – Aids digestion by stimulating and strengthening intestinal peristalsis. Also relieves intestinal spasms, heartburn, colic, flatulence and spasmodic indigestion.

RESPIRATORY SYSTEM – Eases respiratory difficulties and clears the chest by helping to loosen mucus in colds and bronchitis. Soothes the distressing spasms of tickly coughs.

REPRODUCTIVE SYSTEM – Promotes menstruation, good for period pains and leucorrhoea.

NERVOUS SYSTEM – Sedative and tonic to the nerves, effective for states of anxiety and insomnia.

MUSCULAR SYSTEM – Good for muscle spasm and sprains. Especially useful for tired or stiff muscles after strenuous exercise.

EMOTION – Promotes restful sleep and dispels loneliness, grief and all forms of agitation. Marjoram is comforting, warms the emotions and soothes the broken-hearted. Marjoram diminishes the desire for sexual contact. It redirects excessive sexual ardour and reduces obsessive masturbation and nocturnal orgasms while also removing the fear of love.

## Blends:

**DIGESTIVE:**

| marjoram | 6 |
| juniper | 4 |
| anise | 2 |

**RESPIRATORY:**

| marjoram | 6 |
| benzoin | 3 |
| ginger | 3 |

**REPRODUCTIVE:**

| marjoram | 5 |
| sandalwood | 4 |
| sage | 2 |

**NERVOUS:**

| marjoram | 6 |
| rose | 3 |
| lavender | 2 |

**MUSCULAR:**

| marjoram | 7 |
| rosemary | 3 |
| lemongrass | 2 |

**EMOTION:**

| marjoram | 4 |
| frankincense | 2 |
| rose | 2 |

# Melissa

◆◇◆◇◆◇◆◇◆◇◆◇◆◇◆◇◆◇◆◇◆◇◆◇◆◇◆◇◆◇◆◇◆◇◆◇◆◇◆◇

| | |
|---|---|
| **Botanical Name:** | *Melissa officinalis* |
| **Family:** | *Labiatae* |
| **Location:** | Melissa grows mainly in France and Spain. |
| **Extraction:** | Steam distillation of the leaves. |
| **Colour and Odour:** | The essential oil is pale yellow in colour and has a delightful, crisp lemony aroma with a sweet undertone. |
| **Description:** | A small herb growing to about 60 cm with bright green, serrated, slightly wrinkled hairy leaves and yellowish-white flowers. |
| **Background:** | Medicinally important in Europe since medieval times, melissa was considered the 'elixir of life'. It was included in the preparation of a tonic water made in the fourteenth century by the Carmelite nuns in France. Melissa flowers are very attractive to bees, and melissa honey has been prized since ancient times. |
| **Properties:** | Tonic, sedative, calming, antidepressant, antispasmodic, carminative and hypotensive. |
| **Note:** | The yield is extremely low and the genuine oil is very expensive. Consequently, most melissa oil sold commercially is blended with other essential oils. The blended melissa oil may cause irritation in sensitive people. Use in lower concentrations. |

Uses:     DIGESTIVE SYSTEM – Good for vomiting and indigestion of a nervous origin, relieving spasms and flatulence.

CIRCULATORY SYSTEM – A tonic for the heart, slowing its action, relieving palpitations and lowering blood pressure

RESPIRATORY SYSTEM – Useful for colds and influenza.

REPRODUCTIVE SYSTEM – Useful for painful periods.

NERVOUS SYSTEM – Strongly sedative in cases of hysteria and nervous afflictions, especially those related to over-sensitivity, and for constant panic and anxiety.

EMOTION – Melissa is vivacious and provocative, revitalizing the inner self and calming the senses. Makes the heart merry and joyful. Also helpful in dispelling a sense of dejection in times of grief or bereavement. Melissa calms raging emotions, engendering a state of quiet peace.

## Blends:

| DIGESTIVE: | | CIRCULATORY: | | RESPIRATORY: | |
|---|---|---|---|---|---|
| melissa | 5 | melissa | 4 | melissa | 4 |
| peppermint | 3 | ylang-ylang | 4 | ginger | 3 |
| cardamon | 3 | clary sage | 2 | eucalyptus | 3 |

| REPRODUCTIVE: | | NERVOUS: | | EMOTION: | |
|---|---|---|---|---|---|
| melissa | 5 | melissa | 4 | melissa | 4 |
| geranium | 4 | vetivert | 3 | orange | 4 |
| basil | 2 | chamomile (R) | 2 | frankincense | 3 |

# Myrrh

◆ ◇ ◆ ◇ ◆ ◇ ◆ ◇ ◆ ◇ ◆ ◇ ◆ ◇ ◆ ◇ ◆ ◇ ◆ ◇ ◆ ◇ ◆ ◇ ◆ ◇ ◆ ◇ ◆ ◇ ◆ ◇

| | |
|---|---|
| **Botanical Name:** | *Commiphora myrrha* |
| **Family:** | *Burseraceae* |
| **Location:** | The myrrh tree grows in the deserts of northeast Africa and southern Arabia. |
| **Extraction:** | Steam distillation of the gum-resin. |
| **Colour and Odour:** | The essential oil is deep golden-yellow, turning deep amber with age. It has a musty, balsamic, smoky aroma. |
| **Description:** | A small tree with knotted branches, small leaves and white flowers. The resin exudes from natural fissures in the bark and dries on exposure to the air. |
| **Background:** | Myrrh is famous, together with frankincense and gold, as the gifts brought by the three Magi from the East to Jesus when he was born. It is mentioned several times in the Bible. Myrrh was an important ingredient in the famous perfume 'megaleion' of ancient Greece. |
| **Properties:** | Antiseptic, cooling, tonic, stimulant, expectorant, vulnerary, emmenagogic, anti-inflammatory, sedative and astringent. |

**Uses:** RESPIRATORY SYSTEM – A very good expectorant, of value in coughs, bronchitis, colds and flu, especially when there is an excess of thick mucus. An excellent remedy for throat and mouth inflammations and ulcers.

134

SKIN – Cooling on the skin, myrrh is good for mature skin, helping to preserve a youthful complexion. Very useful in a hot, dry climate. Promotes healing in wounds and reduces inflammation. Good for cracked and chapped skin.

EMOTION – The mysterious and seductive qualities of myrrh awaken an awareness of the spiritual reality behind everyday existence. The resultant expanded awareness calms fears and uncertainties about the future. Amplifies strength and courage. Useful for treating states of agitation, restlessness and emotional over-reaction. Cools heated emotions.

## Blends:

| RESPIRATORY: | | SKIN: | | EMOTION: | |
|---|---|---|---|---|---|
| myrrh | 6 | myrrh | 5 | myrrh | 5 |
| eucalyptus | 4 | frankincense | 3 | rose | 4 |
| thyme | 2 | lavender | 2 | lemon | 3 |

# Neroli

| | |
|---|---|
| **Botanical Name:** | *Citrus aurantium* |
| **Family:** | *Rutaceae* |
| **Location:** | Neroli is produced mainly in Egypt, France, Morocco and Tunisia. |
| **Extraction:** | Steam distillation or solvent extraction of the bitter orange flowers. |
| **Colour and Odour:** | The essential oil is pale yellow in colour with an exquisite sweet floral aroma. |
| **Description:** | The bitter orange tree is a small evergreen very similar to the sweet orange tree, although hardier. It has shiny leaves and bears fragrant white flowers. |
| **Background:** | The bitter orange tree is native to China and was introduced to Europe by the Portuguese in the twelfth century. The orange flower was named after the Italian Princess Anne-Marie, Countess of Neroli, who used it to perfume her bath water. It is now considered among the finest perfumery ingredients and is particularly important in Eau-de-Cologne toilet water. The flowers are popularly used in bridal bouquets as they symbolize innocence and fertility. |
| **Properties:** | Sedative, antidepressant, soothing, carminative, antispasmodic and aphrodisiac. |

Uses:   DIGESTIVE SYSTEM – Soothes intestinal spasms and colic.

CIRCULATORY SYSTEM – Slows down the heart rate, therefore useful for cardiac spasms and palpitations.

NERVOUS SYSTEM – Calms and slows the mind; useful for insomnia, hysteria and all states of anxiety and depression.

SKIN – Beneficial for all skin types, especially if there is dryness, redness or irritation. Neroli stimulates the regeneration of new cells and the elimination of old ones, improving skin's elasticity. Generally helpful for all kinds of skin problems such as thread veins, scarring and stretch marks.

EMOTION – Calms highly charged emotional states and helps sufferers to deal with anxieties and fears, bestowing confidence. Rather hypnotic and euphoric for countering states of hysteria. Neroli is a valuable remedy for shock and the disorders caused by shock.

## Blends:

DIGESTIVE:
neroli         5
orange         4
peppermint     2

CIRCULATORY:
neroli          5
ylang-ylang     4
chamomile (R)   2

NERVOUS:
neroli          5
chamomile (R)   3
petitgrain      2

SKIN:
neroli          3
frankincense    2
chamomile (R)   2

EMOTION:
neroli    4
lemon     3
basil     2

# Niaouli

| | |
|---|---|
| **Botanical Name:** | *Melaleuca viridiflora* |
| **Family:** | *Myrtaceae* |
| **Location:** | Niaouli grows in Australia and New Caledonia. |
| **Extraction:** | Steam distillation of the leaves. |
| **Colour and Odour:** | The essential oil is colourless and has a strong, camphorous aroma. |
| **Description:** | A large tree with bushy foliage and yellow flowers. |
| **Background:** | Introduced into European use by the French, niaouli is used in several French hospital wards for its antiseptic properties. |
| **Properties:** | Antiseptic, anti-inflammatory, analgesic, expectorant and tonic. |

**Uses:** RESPIRATORY SYSTEM – Good for all types of pulmonary tract infections such as colds, flu, coughs, sinusitis, laryngitis and bronchitis.

SKIN – Suitable for cleaning minor wounds, cuts, grazes and burns. Also good for treating acne and boils.

EMOTION – Good for treating mental fatigue and confusion.

**Blends:**

| RESPIRATORY: | | SKIN: | | EMOTION: | |
|---|---|---|---|---|---|
| niaouli | 7 | niaouli | 3 | niaouli | 7 |
| pine | 3 | bergamot | 2 | petitgrain | 3 |
| hyssop | 2 | lavender | 2 | rosemary | 2 |

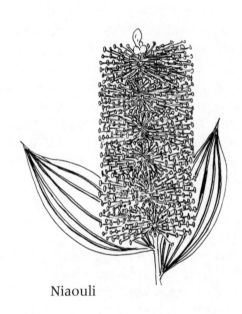

Niaouli

# Nutmeg

◆◇◆◇◆◇◆◇◆◇◆◇◆◇◆◇◆◇◆◇◆◇◆◇◆◇◆◇◆◇◆◇◆◇◆◇◆◇

| | |
|---|---|
| **Botanical Name:** | *Myristica fragans* |
| **Family:** | *Myristicaceae* |
| **Location:** | Nutmeg grows in Grenada, Indonesia and Sri Lanka. |
| **Extraction:** | Steam distillation of the dried kernel (nut). |
| **Colour and Odour:** | The essential oil is clear with a hint of yellow. It has a sharp, warm and spicy aroma. |
| **Description:** | An evergreen tropical tree growing to a height of 12 m. Each male tree can pollinate up to 20 female trees, bearing peach-like fruits. The kernels are sold after drying as nutmeg spice. Surrounding the kernel is a layer of a reddish fleshy covering that is sold separately as the mace spice. Both can be used for extracting essential oils. |
| **Background:** | First mentioned in Europe in the fifth century, nutmeg was traded by the Arabs and was important during the Middle Ages for various medicinal purposes. From 1605 until 1768 the Dutch took over the monopoly of nutmeg production, after which time production reverted back to Indonesia. |
| **Properties:** | Warming, tonic, stimulant and digestive. |
| **Precaution:** | This oil is best used in lower concentrations as it may be over-stimulating. |

Uses:    DIGESTIVE SYSTEM – Encourages appetite and stimulates digestion. Good for nausea, vomiting, flatulence and bad breath.

RESPIRATORY SYSTEM – Helps to strengthen the body against colds.

REPRODUCTIVE SYSTEM – A uterine tonic, helping to regulate scanty periods and to soothe painful ones.

MUSCULAR SYSTEM – Useful for warming and toning the muscles and relieving rheumatic pain.

EMOTION – Helps to disperse nervous anxieties, invigorating and activating the mind. Nutmeg has reputed aphrodisiac properties, being soft, sultry, evocative and seductive. It is gently provocative, arousing and lingering.

## Blends:

**DIGESTIVE:**

| nutmeg | 5 |
|---|---|
| orange | 4 |
| cardamon | 3 |

**RESPIRATORY:**

| nutmeg | 5 |
|---|---|
| benzoin | 4 |
| pine | 2 |

**REPRODUCTIVE:**

| nutmeg | 5 |
|---|---|
| clary sage | 3 |
| geranium | 3 |

**MUSCULAR:**

| nutmeg | 6 |
|---|---|
| B pepper | 4 |
| lavender | 2 |

**EMOTION:**

| nutmeg | 5 |
|---|---|
| bergamot | 4 |
| ylang-ylang | 2 |

# Orange

◆ ◇ ◆ ◇ ◆ ◇ ◆ ◇ ◆ ◇ ◆ ◇ ◆ ◇ ◆ ◇ ◆ ◇ ◆ ◇ ◆ ◇ ◆ ◇ ◆ ◇ ◆ ◇ ◆ ◇

| | |
|---|---|
| **Botanical Name:** | *Citrus sinensis* |
| **Family:** | *Rutaceae* |
| **Location:** | Orange is now widely cultivated for its fruit and juice all around the Mediterranean and in California and Florida. |
| **Extraction:** | Expression of the peel. |
| **Colour and Odour:** | The essential oil is golden yellow in colour and has a sweet, fruity aroma. |
| **Description:** | The sweet orange is produced by a small evergreen tree which is less hardy than the bitter orange tree. It has shiny leaves, white flowers and round fruits. |
| **Background:** | A native of China, the sweet orange was introduced into Europe in the eighteenth century, where it flourished. Orange is a traditional ingredient in mulled wine; pierced with cloves and dried, the fruit is a popular pomander. |
| **Properties:** | Antidepressant, antispasmodic, stomachic and sedative. |

**Uses:**   DIGESTIVE SYSTEM – Promotes peristalsis, easing constipation.

CIRCULATORY SYSTEM – Valuable for treating cardiac spasm or palpitations and reducing blood cholesterol.

EMOTION – Very cheering, joyful, bright and lively,

orange disperses gloomy thoughts, emotional tangles, obsessions and a fear of the unknown, creating a positive outlook. It dispels depression and sadness.

## Blends:

| DIGESTIVE: | | CIRCULATORY: | | EMOTION: | |
|---|---|---|---|---|---|
| orange | 7 | orange | 7 | orange | 7 |
| B pepper | 3 | ylang-ylang | 3 | neroli | 3 |
| peppermint | 2 | lavender | 2 | cinnamon | 2 |

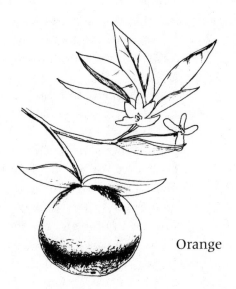

Orange

# Palmarosa

| | |
|---|---|
| **Botanical Name:** | *Cymbopogon martinii* |
| **Family:** | *Graminae* |
| **Location:** | Palmarosa is grown in Africa, Brazil, Comores, India, Indonesia and Pakistan. |
| **Extraction:** | Steam distillation of the dried leaves. |
| **Colour and Odour:** | The essential oil is clear with a hint of yellow. It has a fresh sweet rosy aroma. |
| **Description:** | A wild growing grass with long slender leaves and terminal flowering tops. It has a spreading habit, flourishing in the tropics. |
| **Background:** | Known locally in India as 'rosha', two varieties are cultivated: motia and sofia. The odour of palmarosa resembles rose and geranium essential oils, and is used as a cheaper substitute for scenting soap as well as flavouring tobacco. Formerly, palmarosa oil was shipped to Bulgaria via Constantinople and used to adulterate rose oil, which was produced there. |
| **Properties:** | Tonic, stimulant, antiseptic, cytophylactic, antirheumatic and antidepressant. |

**Uses:**

MUSCULAR SYSTEM – Useful for stiff muscles.
SKIN – Promotes sebum production for dry skin; palmarosa is also good for wrinkles. Encourages skin renewal by aiding cellular regeneration.

Palmarosa is an antiseptic that is beneficial for
skin infections, including acne.

EMOTION – Palmarosa's refreshing and compelling
scent calms agitation and clarifies the mind. It lifts
depression and helps with listlessness.

## Blends:

| MUSCULAR: | | SKIN: | | EMOTION: | |
|---|---|---|---|---|---|
| palmarosa | 7 | palmarosa | 4 | palmarosa | 5 |
| rosemary | 3 | lavender | 2 | lemon | 4 |
| coriander | 2 | frankincense | 2 | geranium | 2 |

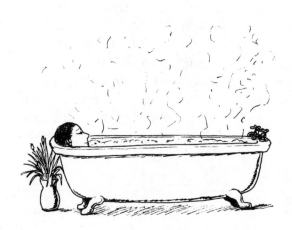

# Parsley

| | |
|---|---|
| **Botanical Name:** | *Petroselinum sativum* |
| **Family:** | *Umbelliferae* |
| **Location:** | Parsley is native to the Mediterranean region and is cultivated in Belgium, France, Germany, Holland, Hungary and India. |
| **Extraction:** | Steam distillation of the seeds. |
| **Colour and Odour:** | The essential oil is yellow in colour and has a herby, spicy odour. |
| **Description:** | A small herb growing up to 60 cm with either flat or crinkly dark green leaves and yellowish flowers. |
| **Background:** | Known to the ancient Greeks and Romans, parsley later became popular in Europe during the sixteenth century for both culinary and medicinal purposes. Well known for its ability to remove the smell of garlic and onions. |
| **Properties:** | Stimulant, diuretic, tonic, carminative, emmenagogic, antiseptic and antispasmodic. |

**Uses:**    DIGESTIVE SYSTEM – Stimulates appetite; helpful for flatulence, cramps and indigestion.

URINARY SYSTEM – Useful in all urinary tract problems. Its diuretic action makes it valuable for easing oedema.

CIRCULATORY SYSTEM – A tonic for the blood vessels; helpful for haemorrhoids.

REPRODUCTIVE SYSTEM – Parsley is especially helpful for weak, anaemic women with scanty periods.

SKIN – Cleanses the blood, which helps all skin disorders.

EMOTION – Sedative to jangled nerves and fretful minds.

## Blends:

| DIGESTIVE: | | URINARY: | | CIRCULATORY: | |
|---|---|---|---|---|---|
| parsley | 4 | parsley | 5 | parsley | 5 |
| lemon | 4 | juniper | 4 | cypress | 4 |
| peppermint | 3 | fennel | 3 | geranium | 3 |

| REPRODUCTIVE: | | SKIN: | | EMOTION: | |
|---|---|---|---|---|---|
| parsley | 4 | parsley | 4 | parsley | 4 |
| geranium | 3 | lavender | 3 | bergamot | 4 |
| rosemary | 3 | juniper | 3 | rosewood | 3 |

# Patchouli

◆ ◇ ◆ ◇ ◆ ◇ ◆ ◇ ◆ ◇ ◆ ◇ ◆ ◇ ◆ ◇ ◆ ◇ ◆ ◇ ◆ ◇ ◆ ◇ ◆ ◇ ◆ ◇ ◆ ◇ ◆ ◇ ◆ ◇ ◆ ◇ ◆ ◇

| | |
|---|---|
| **Botanical Name:** | *Pogostemon cablin* |
| **Family:** | *Labiatae* |
| **Location:** | Patchouli is cultivated in Brazil, China, India, Indonesia and the Philippines. |
| **Extraction:** | Steam distillation of the dried leaves after fermentation. |
| **Colour and Odour:** | The essential oil is deep amber in colour with a persistent, musty, earthy and exotic aroma that is also very penetrating. This essential oil improves with age. |
| **Description:** | A bushy plant growing to about 90 cm with broad oval-shaped leaves and purplish flowers. |
| **Background:** | Patchouli has long been prized for its strong scent. Used to scent shawls in India, this practice was copied by Paisley weavers after patchouli was introduced to Britain in 1820. It is important in perfumery as an excellent fixative. Patchouli was very popular as a personal scent in England during the 'psychedelic' sixties. |
| **Properties:** | Sedative, tonic, cytophylactic, anti-inflammatory and nervine. |

**Uses:** NERVOUS SYSTEM – Of value in nervous debility, strengthening the nerves.
SKIN – Treats cracked skin and weeping sores, having mild anti-inflammatory properties. Also

suitable for skin allergies. Patchouli is rejuvenating and is good for mature skin, promoting the growth of new skin cells and helping skin to maintain suppleness.

EMOTION – Patchouli has a sedative effect useful in anxiety states. The profoundly earthy smell of patchouli can also stimulate the nervous system. Its penetrating quality is very forceful, reaching deep into the emotions, with voluptuous suggestions shaking one out of a sense of indifference and neglect. Dispels feelings of anxiety about sex.

## Blends:

| NERVOUS: | | SKIN: | | EMOTION: | |
|---|---|---|---|---|---|
| patchouli | 5 | patchouli | 3 | patchouli | 5 |
| rose | 4 | neroli | 2 | orange | 4 |
| neroli | 2 | sandalwood | 2 | geranium | 2 |

# Peppermint

◆ ◇ ◆ ◇ ◆ ◇ ◆ ◇ ◆ ◇ ◆ ◇ ◆ ◇ ◆ ◇ ◆ ◇ ◆ ◇ ◆ ◇ ◆ ◇ ◆ ◇ ◆ ◇ ◆ ◇ ◆ ◇

**Botanical Name:** *Mentha piperita*

**Family:** *Labiatae*

**Location:** Peppermint grows throughout Europe and is now largely cultivated in the United States, which is the major world producer.

**Extraction:** Steam distillation of the leaves.

**Colour and Odour:** The essential oil is colourless and has a strongly piercing, sharp aroma.

**Description:** A small herb growing up to 90 cm, it has dark green leaves with serrated edges and small purplish flowers. The plant propagates by underground runners and prefers to grow in damp places.

**Background:** The plant is named after Mentha, a nymph much loved by Pluto in Greek mythology. Persephone, Pluto's wife, was so jealous of Mentha that she trod her into the ground. Pluto, however, turned her into the enchanting herb we all know so well. Peppermint oil is used medicinally to treat irritable bowel syndrome. The aroma of the oil is very strong and may counteract homoeopathic remedies. It is also strongly disliked by pests, both rodents and insects.

**Properties:** Analgesic, sedative, antiseptic, anti-inflammatory, expectorant, antispasmodic and sudorific.

**Uses:**　DIGESTIVE SYSTEM – A prime remedy for all
digestive disorders including indigestion, colic,
heartburn, flatulence, diarrhoea, bloating,
stomach pains, nausea and vomiting.
RESPIRATORY SYSTEM – Ideal for most types of
colds and influenza, especially sinus congestion,
dry cough and sore throat. Also effective in the
treatment of bronchitis and pneumonia.
REPRODUCTIVE SYSTEM – Very good for
dysmenorrhoea, scanty periods and breast
congestion.
NERVOUS SYSTEM – Valuable in many nervous
disorders such as headache, hysteria, palpitations,
trembling and paralysis.
SKIN – Relieves any kind of skin irritation or
itching and rashes. A good remedy for chilblains.
EMOTION – Aids concentration and memory.
Stimulates the brain to think clearly, encouraging
a fresh and bright feeling. Excellent for mental
fatigue and depression. Peppermint is a good
remedy for shock. Emotionally, it dispels feelings
of inferiority as well as those of pride and egoism.

## Blends:

**DIGESTIVE:**

| | |
|---|---|
| peppermint | 5 |
| ginger | 4 |
| lavender | 3 |

**RESPIRATORY:**

| | |
|---|---|
| peppermint | 5 |
| sandalwood | 4 |
| pine | 3 |

**REPRODUCTIVE:**

| | |
|---|---|
| peppermint | 5 |
| geranium | 4 |
| rosemary | 3 |

**NERVOUS:**

| | |
|---|---|
| peppermint | 5 |
| lavender | 4 |
| chamomile (R) | 3 |

**SKIN:**

| | |
|---|---|
| peppermint | 4 |
| lavender | 2 |
| chamomile (R) | 2 |

**EMOTION:**

| | |
|---|---|
| peppermint | 4 |
| lemon | 4 |
| lavender | 2 |

# Petitgrain

◆ ◇ ◆ ◇ ◆ ◇ ◆ ◇ ◆ ◇ ◆ ◇ ◆ ◇ ◆ ◇ ◆ ◇ ◆ ◇ ◆ ◇ ◆ ◇ ◆ ◇ ◆ ◇ ◆ ◇ ◆ ◇

| | |
|---|---|
| **Botanical Name:** | *Citrus aurantium* |
| **Family:** | *Rutaceae* |
| **Location:** | Petitgrain is now produced from bitter orange trees in Africa, Haiti and Paraguay. |
| **Extraction:** | Steam distillation of the leaves and twigs. |
| **Colour and Odour:** | The essential oil is colourless with a hint of yellow. It has a fresh, invigorating fragrance with a sweet herbaceous under tone. |
| **Description:** | Petitgrain is obtained from the bitter orange tree, as is neroli. |
| **Background:** | The essential oil of petitgrain was formerly distilled from the small (cherry-sized), unripened fruits of the orange tree. This practice reduced the yield of the mature fruits, so petitgrain oil is now obtained from the leaves and twigs of the orange tree. It is an important ingredient in the original Eau de Cologne toilet water. |
| **Properties:** | Sedative, antidepressant, antispasmodic, antiseptic, digestive, nervine, stimulant and tonic. |

**Uses:** NERVOUS SYSTEM – Sedative effect calms the nerves and aids insomnia.

SKIN – Good for irritated or spotty skin.

EMOTION – Petitgrain promotes mental clarity, preparing the intellect for further work by

sharpening the thought processes. It strengthens
the emotionally delicate, restoring faith and
calming the anger of those experiencing a sense
of betrayal.

**Blends:**

| NERVOUS: | | SKIN: | | EMOTION: | |
|---|---|---|---|---|---|
| petitgrain | 7 | petitgrain | 3 | petitgrain | 6 |
| lavender | 2 | geranium | 2 | juniper | 3 |
| chamomile (R) | 2 | bergamot | 2 | orange | 3 |

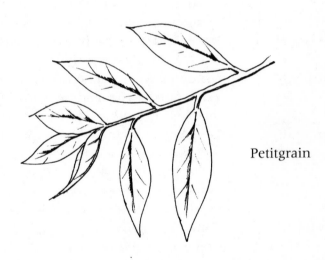

Petitgrain

# Pine

♦◇♦◇♦◇♦◇♦◇♦◇♦◇♦◇♦◇♦◇♦◇♦◇♦◇♦◇♦◇♦◇♦◇♦◇♦◇♦◇

| | |
|---|---|
| **Botanical Name:** | *Pinus sylvestris* |
| **Family:** | *Pinaceae* |
| **Location:** | Pine grows in northern Europe and Russia. |
| **Extraction:** | Steam distillation of the needles (leaves). |
| **Colour and Odour:** | The essential oil is colourless with a strong, fresh and penetrating aroma. |
| **Description:** | A large evergreen conifer tree growing up to 40 m and having a reddish, deeply fissured bark and long stiff needle-like leaves with pointed, brown, woody cones. The tree exhales its essential oil into the surrounding atmosphere; it is an exhilarating experience to walk through a pine forest breathing in the crisp fragrance. |
| **Background:** | Long known to the ancients, pine is now important for producing timber and turpentine. Its medicinal value was known to the Arabs, Greeks and Romans. An excellent air freshener and disinfectant. |
| **Properties:** | Refreshing, deodorant, strongly antiseptic, expectorant and stimulant. |

**Uses:**     RESPIRATORY SYSTEM – Very good for colds, catarrh and sore throats. Eases breathlessness and helps to clear the sinuses. Pine is especially helpful for hay fever. (Recommended for use in the sauna.)

MUSCULAR SYSTEM – Relieves muscular or

rheumatic pain and general stiffness.

EMOTION – Pine cleanses the negative vibes picked up in crowded places and is invigorating, promoting feelings of energy and well-being. Helps with loss of concentration, mental fatigue and emotional weakness. Invigorates the apathetic and depressed, re-activating their energy.

## Blends:

| RESPIRATORY: | | MUSCULAR: | | EMOTION: | |
|---|---|---|---|---|---|
| pine | 6 | pine | 6 | pine | 5 |
| eucalyptus | 4 | rosemary | 4 | juniper | 4 |
| sandalwood | 2 | B pepper | 4 | basil | 2 |

# Rose

◆ ◇ ◆ ◇ ◆ ◇ ◆ ◇ ◆ ◇ ◆ ◇ ◆ ◇ ◆ ◇ ◆ ◇ ◆ ◇ ◆ ◇ ◆ ◇ ◆ ◇ ◆ ◇ ◆ ◇ ◆ ◇ ◆ ◇ ◆ ◇

| | |
|---|---|
| **Botanical Name:** | *Rosa damascena* (damask rose); *Rosa centifolia* (cabbage rose). |
| **Family:** | *Rosaceae* |
| **Location:** | Rose otto and rose absolute have long been produced at the perfume centre in Grasse, in southern France. Other countries of production include Egypt, Morocco and Turkey. However, the finest rose otto is produced in Bulgaria. |
| **Extraction:** | The otto is distilled from damask rose; the absolute is solvent-extracted from the cabbage rose. Both the otto and the absolute are extremely expensive but very useful in aromatherapy. |
| **Colour and Odour:** | The otto is pale yellow in colour and has a sweet, rich, deep floral-spicy aroma; the absolute is dark amber in colour with a sweet, tenacious floral scent. |
| **Description:** | A small prickly shrub growing to about 90 cm–1.8 m high with flowers that have an exquisite fragrance. The flowers are picked very early in the morning for both distillation and solvent extraction. |
| **Background:** | One of the oldest and best known of all perfumes. The rose is also the most loved, praised, sought-after and written about of all flowers.<br><br>The history of rose otto is traditionally |

traced to the wedding of the Mogul Emperor Djihanguyr and Princess Nour Djihan in India. When rose petals were placed on the water of the canals surrounding the palace, it was noticed that a thin film of oil was left floating on the surface of the water. On closer examination this substance was found to smell of roses. Distillation of rose otto apparently started shortly thereafter, both in India and also in neighbouring Persia. In modern times the Indian and Persian rose otto production has declined and the modern production of rose otto is found centred around the Mediterranean lands. The amount of oil in the rose is so small that it requires 6,000 roses to produce 30 ml of otto. Rose oil is therefore one of the most expensive of all perfume ingredients.

**Properties:** Cleansing, tonic, soothing, antidepressant, aphrodisiac, antiseptic, anti-inflammatory and choleretic.

**Uses:** DIGESTIVE SYSTEM – Strengthens the stomach and promotes the flow of bile; useful in the treatment of jaundice.

CIRCULATORY SYSTEM – Tones the blood vessels, cleanses the blood, promotes circulation, relieves cardiac congestion and regulates the action of the heart. Good for anaemia.

REPRODUCTIVE SYSTEM – Cleanses the womb, regulates menstrual function; useful in the treatment of impotence and sterility. Eases premenstrual tension and painful periods.

NERVOUS SYSTEM – Rose's soothing action on the nerves promotes sleep.

SKIN – Useful for all skin types but particularly so for mature, dry or sensitive skin with any redness or inflammation. Rose's tonic and astringent effect on the capillaries helps to reduce thread veins. Rejuvenates and regenerates the skin.

EMOTION – Rose is luxurious and erotically sensual. It provides emotional comfort in times of turbulence, enlivens the heart, boosts confidence and brings out one's deepest feelings, increasing affection and sexual desire. The scent calms strife and instils a feeling of peace and happiness, ensuring warm, happy associations. It soothes and calms hyperactive personalities who are ill at ease, unsettled, unsure or unhappy with themselves or who feel a sense of guilt, jealousy, grief and resentment.

## Blends:

**DIGESTIVE:**

| | |
|---|---|
| rose | 5 |
| orange | 4 |
| peppermint | 2 |

**CIRCULATORY:**

| | |
|---|---|
| rose | 6 |
| rosemary | 2 |
| melissa | 2 |

**REPRODUCTIVE:**

| | |
|---|---|
| rose | 6 |
| sandalwood | 5 |
| geranium | 2 |

**NERVOUS:**

| | |
|---|---|
| rose | 6 |
| chamomile (R) | 2 |
| frankincense | 2 |

**SKIN:**

| | |
|---|---|
| rose | 3 |
| lavender | 2 |
| patchouli | 2 |

**EMOTION:**

| | |
|---|---|
| rose | 5 |
| mandarin | 4 |
| cedarwood | 2 |

Very old are the woods;
And the buds that break
Out of the briar's boughs,
When March winds break
So old with their beauty are –
Oh! no man knows
Though what wild centuries
Roves back the rose.

*Walter de la Mare*

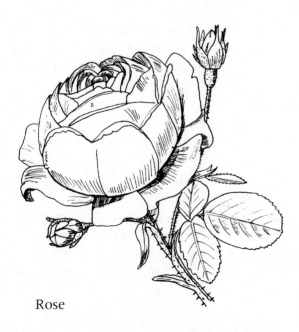

Rose

# Rosemary

◆ ◇ ◆ ◇ ◆ ◇ ◆ ◇ ◆ ◇ ◆ ◇ ◆ ◇ ◆ ◇ ◆ ◇ ◆ ◇ ◆ ◇ ◆ ◇ ◆ ◇ ◆ ◇ ◆ ◇ ◆ ◇ ◆ ◇ ◆ ◇ ◆ ◇

| | |
|---|---|
| **Botanical Name:** | *Rosmarinus officinalis* |
| **Family:** | *Labiatae* |
| **Location:** | Rosemary is cultivated in the Balkan States, England, France, Morocco, Portugal, Russia, Spain and Tunisia. |
| **Extraction:** | Steam distillation of the leaves. |
| **Colour and Odour:** | The essential oil is colourless and has a warm, sharp, refreshing and camphorous aroma. |
| **Description:** | A small shrub growing to about 90 cm high, it has long, straight stems, narrow, pointed leaves about 2.5 cm long, and small, pale blue flowers. |
| **Background:** | Important as an ingredient in a famous toilet water produced in 1370 and named 'Hungary Water' after Queen Elizabeth of Hungary, who was reputed to have retained her beautiful appearance into old age. Rosemary is also one of the ingredients in the classic Eau-de-Cologne. |
| **Properties:** | Stimulant, antispasmodic, carminative, stomachic, tonic, astringent, cleansing, cephalic, cordial, diuretic and nervine. |

**Uses:**    DIGESTIVE SYSTEM – Useful for indigestion, stomach pains, colitis, flatulence and constipation. Rosemary is also a good remedy for hepatic disorders such as jaundice, hepatitis, cirrhosis, gallstones and bile duct blockage, being tonic to the liver and gall-bladder.

URINARY SYSTEM – Rosemary promotes the flow of urine, thus helping alleviate water retention.

CIRCULATORY SYSTEM – Stimulating effect on the heart; promotes circulation and helps to improve eyesight. Normalizes poor circulation and low blood pressure, being an excellent heart tonic. Good for palpitations and hardening of the arteries.

RESPIRATORY SYSTEM – Useful for colds, influenza and chronic bronchitis with associated coughs.

REPRODUCTIVE SYSTEM – Good for menstrual cramps and scanty periods.

NERVOUS SYSTEM – Stimulant and tonic to the nerves and useful for all nervous disorders and impairment of sensitivity as well as hysteria and paralysis. Good for headaches, mental fatigue, nervous exhaustion and debility.

MUSCULAR SYSTEM – Very good for rheumatic and muscular pain, especially tired, stiff and over worked muscles. Rosemary warms cold limbs, especially during winter, and is particularly good for rheumatism brought on by the cold.

SKIN – A good skin tonic. Rosemary stimulates the scalp and promotes hair growth. Excellent for scalp problems such as dandruff, greasy hair and hair loss.

EMOTION – Clears the mind of confusion and doubt and promotes mental clarity. Rosemary stimulates sensitivity and increases creativity by lifting exhaustion and awakening the heart.

**Blends:**

| DIGESTIVE: | | URINARY: | | CIRCULATORY: | |
|---|---|---|---|---|---|
| rosemary | 7 | rosemary | 7 | rosemary | 6 |
| B pepper | 3 | marjoram | 3 | frankincense | 4 |
| fennel | 2 | clary sage | 2 | melissa | 2 |

| RESPIRATORY: | | REPRODUCTIVE: | | NERVOUS: | |
|---|---|---|---|---|---|
| rosemary | 6 | rosemary | 6 | rosemary | 6 |
| benzoin | 3 | jasmine | 4 | basil | 4 |
| cajeput | 3 | parsley | 2 | lavender | 2 |

| MUSCULAR: | | SKIN: | | EMOTION: | |
|---|---|---|---|---|---|
| rosemary | 7 | rosemary | 7 | rosemary | 5 |
| B pepper | 4 | bay | 3 | bergamot | 3 |
| ginger | 2 | cypress | 2 | grapefruit | 3 |

A decoction of rosemary in wine helps cold diseases of the head and brain such as giddiness and swimmings, drowsiness or dullness, the dumb palsy, loss of speech, lethargy and falling sickness. It is both drunk and the temples bathed with it.

It eases pains in the teeth and gums and is comfortable to the stomach. It is a remedy for windiness in the stomach, bowels and spleen, and powerfully expels it. Both flowers and leaves are profitable for the whites if taken daily. The leaves used in ointments, or infused in oil, help benumbed joints, sinews, or members.

The oil of rosemary is a sovereign help for all the diseases mentioned. Touch the temples and nostrils with two or three drops or take one to three drops for inward diseases. But use discretion, for it is quick and piercing, and only a little must be taken at a time.

*Nicholas Culpeper*

Rosemary

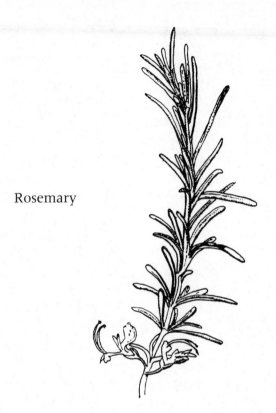

# Rosewood (and Ho Leaf)

| | |
|---|---|
| **Botanical Name:** | *Aniba rosaeodora* |
| **Family:** | *Lauraceae* |
| **Location:** | Rosewood is obtained mainly from Brazil, and formerly also from French Guyana. |
| **Extraction:** | Steam distillation of the heartwood chippings. |
| **Colour and Odour:** | The essential oil is colourless and has a woody middle note and floral undertone. The odour is rich and subtle. |
| **Description:** | A tree growing profusely up to 37.5 m in the tropical rainforests of the Amazon. The logs are cut and floated downriver during the flood season between April and July. |
| **Background:** | Rosewood oil has only recently been introduced to the aromatherapy repertoire. The rose-scented wood is used to make cabinets. It was probably used by the native Indians in the Amazon jungle for medicinal purposes. |
| **Note:** | An alternative to rosewood oil is ho leaf oil, obtained from *Cinnamomum camphora*, a tree growing in China. Both oils share the same properties and can be used for treating the same problems. |
| **Properties:** | Tonic, stimulant and sedative, slightly analgesic, antidepressant, cephalic (head-clearing), deodorant, antiseptic and tonic. |

**Uses:**    NERVOUS SYSTEM – For clearing headaches resulting from nausea, gently relieving the effects of nervousness and stress. Also for steadying the nerves during stressful periods such as examinations, job interviews or crisis situations.
SKIN – Promotes cellular regeneration. Valuable for wrinkles, ageing, sensitive or inflamed skins.
EMOTION – Emotionally uplifting and enlivening, stabilizing the nervous system. It has an overall calming effect without causing any drowsiness. Helpful when weary and over-burdened. Particularly valuable during meditation, and helps daydreamers to concentrate. Its subtle but real aphrodisiac properties are helpful in treating mood swings and emotional confusion and reviving the libido. Induces a warm and comforting feeling for counteracting feelings of neglect, abandonment and paranoia. Useful for clearing the atmosphere or recharging your energy. Rosewood produces tranquility while exhilarating the consciousness.

## Blends:

| NERVOUS: | | SKIN: | | EMOTION: | |
|---|---|---|---|---|---|
| rosewood | 6 | rosewood | 3 | rosewood | 6 |
| basil | 3 | frankincense | 2 | orange | 3 |
| lavender | 2 | sandalwood | 2 | coriander | 2 |

# Sage

◆ ◇ ◆ ◇ ◆ ◇ ◆ ◇ ◆ ◇ ◆ ◇ ◆ ◇ ◆ ◇ ◆ ◇ ◆ ◇ ◆ ◇ ◆ ◇ ◆ ◇ ◆ ◇ ◆ ◇ ◆ ◇ ◆ ◇ ◆ ◇

| | |
|---|---|
| **Botanical Name:** | *Salvia officinalis* |
| **Family:** | *Labiatae* |
| **Location:** | Sage grows in the Mediterranean region and is cultivated in Albania, France, Greece, Italy and Turkey. |
| **Extraction:** | Steam distillation of the leaves. |
| **Colour and Odour:** | The essential oil is colourless with a fresh, warm, herbaceous and camphoraceous aroma. |
| **Description:** | A herb reaching about 60 cm and having greyish-green leaves and bluish flowers. |
| **Background:** | Long thought to prolong life and promote wisdom, sage remained very popular throughout Europe, often used as a tea (indeed, it still is, though less commonly). The Chinese have long regarded sage very highly and at the height of the tea trade would barter 3 kg of their own tea for a 1 kg of sage. |
| **Properties:** | Tonic, antispasmodic, antiseptic, digestive, emmenagogue and astringent. |
| **Precaution:** | This oil is best used in lower concentrations as it may cause irritation in sensitive people. |

Uses:     DIGESTIVE SYSTEM – Helpful for weak or
debilitated digestion, also good for diarrhoea.
RESPIRATORY SYSTEM – Strengthens the lungs and

is useful for colds, flu, coughs and sore throats.

REPRODUCTIVE SYSTEM – Promotes menstruation and is helpful for scanty periods or menstrual cramps. Eases hot flushes and sweating during the menopause.

MUSCULAR SYSTEM – Relaxes the muscles, especially when they have been overworked as in weight-training or other strenuous sports.

SKIN – Good for cuts and wounds.

EMOTION – Quickens the senses, strengthens the memory and tones the conscious mind. Indicated for tiredness, depression and grief.

## Blends:

| DIGESTIVE: | | RESPIRATORY: | | REPRODUCTIVE: | |
|---|---|---|---|---|---|
| sage | 6 | sage | 5 | sage | 6 |
| peppermint | 4 | eucalyptus | 4 | geranium | 3 |
| orange | 2 | thyme | 2 | cypress | 3 |
| | | | | | |
| MUSCULAR: | | SKIN: | | EMOTION: | |
| sage | 7 | sage | 3 | sage | 4 |
| rosemary | 3 | lavender | 2 | bergamot | 2 |
| marjoram | 2 | chamomile (R) | 2 | lime | 2 |

# Sandalwood

◆◇◆◇◆◇◆◇◆◇◆◇◆◇◆◇◆◇◆◇◆◇◆◇◆◇◆◇◆◇◆◇◆◇◆◇◆◇

**Botanical Name:** *Santalum album*
**Family:** *Santalaceae*
**Location:** Sandalwood essential oil is produced in India and is now a monopoly of the Indian government.
**Extraction:** Steam distillation of the heartwood.
**Colour and Odour:** The essential oil is pale yellow in colour and has a very persistent, sweet woody base note with a delicate, spicy, oriental undertone. There are certain individuals who have difficulty smelling this oil.
**Description:** The sandalwood tree is a small and slow growing evergreen, reaching about 6–9 m in about 20–30 years in the forests in India. It is parasitic, growing upon other trees. Only very mature trees are cut down; the logs are then left for termites to remove the sapwood, leaving the fragrant heartwood.
**Background:** Sandalwood has a long history of use in India, being mentioned in the earliest medical texts. It was also widely used as incense in religious ceremonies; the wood would be burned at funerals as it was believed to help free the soul. It is an important perfume and cosmetic ingredient. As a perfume, sandalwood is very long lasting and is used as a fixative

for other perfume ingredients. A variety of wooden articles and furniture are made from the fragrant heartwood. The Chinese import large quantities of sandalwood for medicinal use.

**Properties:** Tonic, emollient, sedative, anti-inflammatory and expectorant.

**Uses:** URINARY SYSTEM – Antiseptic for all urinary disorders.

RESPIRATORY SYSTEM – Very useful for chronic bronchitis, laryngitis, sore throat, hiccups and dry coughs.

REPRODUCTIVE SYSTEM – Good for leucorrhoea.

IMMUNE SYSTEM – Stimulates the spleen, promotes white blood cell production and strengthens the immune system against infection.

SKIN – Good for all skin types, especially dry or dehydrated skin.

EMOTION – Sweet, warm and rich, sandalwood is profoundly seductive and a true aphrodisiac, dispelling anxiety and depression. Casts out cynicism and obsessional attitudes, especially strong ties with the past, effecting a cure in cases of sexual dysfunction. Long used as an aid to meditation to help focus the mind away from distracting chatter and create the right mood. It stills the soul and allows it to reach the deepest states of meditation, helping to induce a sense of religious union and spirituality. Sandalwood comforts and helps the dying to make peace with the world.

## Blends:

| URINARY: | | RESPIRATORY: | | REPRODUCTIVE: | |
|---|---|---|---|---|---|
| sandalwood | 7 | sandalwood | 7 | sandalwood | 7 |
| juniper | 3 | myrrh | 3 | benzoin | 3 |
| bergamot | 2 | lavender | 2 | rose | 2 |

| IMMUNE: | | SKIN: | | EMOTION: | |
|---|---|---|---|---|---|
| sandalwood | 6 | sandalwood | 4 | sandalwood | 6 |
| tea tree | 4 | chamomile (R) | 2 | rose | 3 |
| lavender | 2 | geranium | 2 | frankincense | 2 |

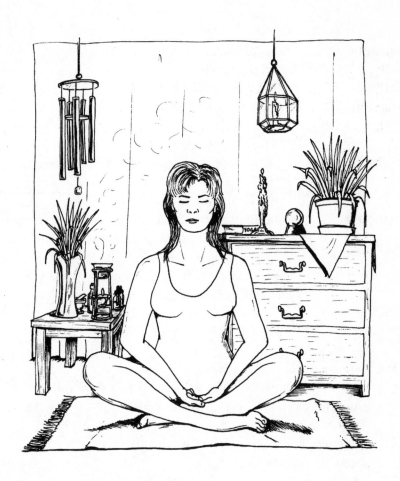

# Tea Tree

◆◇◆◇◆◇◆◇◆◇◆◇◆◇◆◇◆◇◆◇◆◇◆◇◆◇◆◇◆◇◆◇◆◇◆◇◆◇

| | |
|---|---|
| **Botanical Name:** | *Melaleuca alternifolia* |
| **Family:** | *Myrtaceae* |
| **Location:** | Tea tree grows in Australia. |
| **Extraction:** | Steam distillation of the leaves. |
| **Colour and Odour:** | The essential oil is colourless with a fresh, sharp, pungent and camphorous aroma. |
| **Description:** | A small tree with small leaves, growing up to 6 m and found in marshy areas; now cultivated on plantations. |
| **Background:** | Long used by the Australian aborigines for its medicinal properties. It was used by the British colonists as a substitute brew for tea, hence its present name. Tea tree was introduced into European use in 1927. |
| **Properties:** | Antiseptic, antibacterial, anti fungal, stimulant and expectorant. |

**Uses:**     URINARY SYSTEM – Good for cystitis.

RESPIRATORY SYSTEM – Valuable for colds and flu, relieving catarrh and sinusitis.

REPRODUCTIVE SYSTEM – Good for all kinds of vaginal infection such as thrush. Also good for genital and anal itching.

SKIN – Very effective in clearing infected wounds, especially when there is pus. Tea tree is excellent for all types of skin problems, particularly those affecting the feet (such as Athlete's foot, corns, callouses and verrucas). Also good for warts and pierced ear and nail-bed infections. An effective treatment for cold sores, shingles and chicken pox. A good cleanser and deodorizer.

EMOTION – Tea tree is very clarifying and head-clearing, cleansing the imagination of disturbing thoughts.

**Blends:**

URINARY:
tea tree 6
sandalwood 3
myrrh 3

RESPIRATORY:
tea tree 5
pine 3
thyme 2

REPRODUCTIVE:
tea tree 5
myrrh 4
chamomile (R) 3

SKIN:
tea tree 7
eucalyptus 3
bergamot 2

EMOTION:
tea tree 5
juniper 4
frankincense 2

# Thyme

◆◇◆◇◆◇◆◇◆◇◆◇◆◇◆◇◆◇◆◇◆◇◆◇◆◇◆◇◆◇◆◇◆◇

| | |
|---|---|
| **Botanical Name:** | *Thymus vulgaris* |
| **Family:** | *Labiatae* |
| **Location:** | Thyme grows in Algeria, France, Morocco, Israel, Spain, Tunisia and Turkey. |
| **Extraction:** | Steam distillation of the leaves and flowering tops. |
| **Colour and Odour:** | The essential oil is pale yellow in colour with a warm, spicy-herbaceous and powerful aroma. |
| **Description:** | A small bush reaching to about 20 cm high with small greyish-green oval leaves and tiny purplish flowers. |
| **Background:** | Long known to the early Greeks and Romans for its antiseptic properties. Thyme is much used in cooking for its flavour and is popularly grown in the warmer parts of the Mediterranean region. |
| **Note:** | An essential oil of wild thyme which is distilled from *Thymus serpyllum* has similar properties to the essential oil of *Thymus vulgaris*. |
| **Properties:** | Digestive, stimulant, antiseptic, diuretic and expectorant. |
| **Precaution:** | This oil is best used in lower concentrations as it may cause irritation in sensitive people. |

**Uses:**   DIGESTIVE SYSTEM – Helps with sluggish digestion, its antiseptic property valuable in gastric and intestinal infections. Stimulates appetite, especially during convalescence.

URINARY SYSTEM – Thyme is diuretic and is useful for all infections of the bladder and the urinary tract.

CIRCULATORY SYSTEM – Stimulates circulation and raises low blood pressure.

RESPIRATORY SYSTEM – Useful for all respiratory infections including mouth and throat infections. Excellent for removing mucus in cases of both chronic and acute bronchitis.

SKIN – Helpful with wounds, sores, boils and carbuncles. Thyme is a tonic for the scalp.

EMOTION – Cheers the heart, lifts the spirits and promotes courage. The scent prevents nightmares or negative dreams. Very useful for people who tend to indulge in fantasies or daydreams, helping them to focus intellectually.

**Blends:**

| DIGESTIVE: | | URINARY: | | CIRCULATORY: | |
|---|---|---|---|---|---|
| thyme | 5 | thyme | 5 | thyme | 5 |
| bergamot | 5 | celery | 4 | B pepper | 3 |
| chamomile (R) | 2 | juniper | 3 | rosemary | 2 |

| RESPIRATORY: | | SKIN: | | EMOTION: | |
|---|---|---|---|---|---|
| thyme | 5 | thyme | 3 | thyme | 4 |
| myrrh | 3 | tea tree | 2 | grapefruit | 4 |
| sage | 2 | lime | 2 | cedarwood | 3 |

# Vetivert

◆ ◇ ◆ ◇ ◆ ◇ ◆ ◇ ◆ ◇ ◆ ◇ ◆ ◇ ◆ ◇ ◆ ◇ ◆ ◇ ◆ ◇ ◆ ◇ ◆ ◇ ◆ ◇ ◆ ◇ ◆ ◇ ◆ ◇ ◆ ◇

| | |
|---|---|
| **Botanical Name:** | *Vetiveria zizanioides* |
| **Family:** | *Graminae* |
| **Location:** | Vetivert grows in India and Indonesia. |
| **Extraction:** | Steam distillation of the dried roots. |
| **Colour and Odour:** | The essential oil is thick and dark reddish-brown in colour with a deep, smoky and earthy scent. |
| **Description:** | A tall, tufted, perennial tropical grass growing in India. The plant is cultivated for its roots, which are collected for extracting the essential oil. Older roots produce better quality scent, as they improve with age. The rooting system helps to prevent soil erosion, especially during the rainy season. |
| **Background:** | Vetivert has long been used in India for its perfume and insect-repellent properties. It is placed with linen to repel moths. The roots are woven into awnings and blinds and hung on the windows in India, where they emanate their scent on warm days when sprinkled with water. |
| **Properties:** | Sedative, grounding and relaxing. |

Uses:  NERVOUS SYSTEM – Deeply relaxing and good for nervous debility.
SKIN – Useful for mature, dry or irritated skin. Strengthens the connective tissues and promotes skin regeneration.

EMOTION – Protects against oversensitivity and being over-affected by other people's emotions. It can also be used for relieving deeply felt tensions and fears. Settles the nerves of people who are too open and out of balance. Induces tranquility. Its earthy scent is sexually arousing and strengthening.

## Blends:

| NERVOUS: | | SKIN: | | EMOTION: | |
|---|---|---|---|---|---|
| vetivert | 6 | vetivert | 3 | vetivert | 4 |
| rosemary | 3 | rose | 2 | rosewood | 3 |
| petitgrain | 3 | frankincense | 2 | mandarin | 3 |

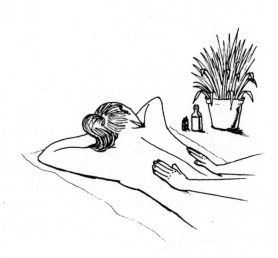

# Ylang-Ylang

| | |
|---|---|
| **Botanical Name:** | *Cananga odorata* |
| **Family:** | *Annonaceae* |
| **Location:** | Ylang-ylang is cultivated in the Comores, Java, Madagascar, the Philippines, Reunion and Sumatra. |
| **Extraction:** | Steam distillation of the flower petals. |
| **Colour and Odour:** | The essential oil is clear with a hint of yellow. It has an intensely sweet and heady scent with an exotic and voluptuous quality. |
| **Description:** | The ylang-ylang tree grows to a height of 7.5–18 m. The flowers are deep yellow in colour with thick petals. These are picked early in the morning for distillation to obtain the essential oil. 'Ylang-ylang' is a Malay word meaning 'flower of flowers'. |
| **Background:** | The flowers are used by the native women in Indonesia to perfume their hair. Ylang-ylang is often mixed with coconut oil; this concoction was sold as the famous 'Macassar' hair oil during the Victorian era. The flowers are also spread on the beds of Indonesian newlyweds on their wedding night. |
| **Properties:** | Evocative, euphoric, sedative, hypotensive and aphrodisiac. |

Uses:   CIRCULATORY SYSTEM – Valuable for reducing high
blood pressure and an abnormally fast heart rate.
RESPIRATORY SYSTEM – Excellent for slowing
down abnormally rapid breathing.
REPRODUCTIVE SYSTEM – Useful in cases of
impotence and frigidity.
NERVOUS SYSTEM – Indicated for stress-related
disorders.
SKIN – Has a soothing effect and is especially good
for the face and for oily skin types. Ylang-ylang
balances the secretion of sebum.
EMOTION – Pacifies the mind, dispelling
stubbornness and anger and creating a feeling of
peace. Dissipates jealousy and soothes frustrations.
Ylang-ylang is excitingly sensuous and is effective
against introversion and emotional coldness,
promoting confidence.

## Blends:

| CIRCULATORY: | | RESPIRATORY: | | REPRODUCTIVE: | |
|---|---|---|---|---|---|
| ylang-ylang | 7 | ylang-ylang | 5 | ylang-ylang | 5 |
| chamomile (R) | 3 | frankincense | 4 | rose | 4 |
| lavender | 2 | cypress | 3 | jasmine | 3 |

| NERVOUS: | | SKIN: | | EMOTION: | |
|---|---|---|---|---|---|
| ylang-ylang | 7 | ylang-ylang | 2 | ylang-ylang | 5 |
| rose | 3 | chamomile (R) | 2 | cedarwood | 5 |
| lavender | 2 | mandarin | 2 | rosewood | 2 |

# Part Three

# Recipes

◆◇◆◇◆◇◆◇◆◇◆◇◆◇◆◇◆◇◆◇◆◇◆◇◆◇◆◇◆◇◆◇◆◇◆◇◆◇◆◇

# ◆ Baths

## Diuretic Baths

| | | | | | | |
|---|---|---|---|---|---|---|
| juniper | 3 | juniper | 3 | rosemary | | 3 |
| rosemary | 3 | fennel | 3 | geranium | | 3 |
| fennel | 2 | lemon | 2 | cypress | | 2 |

## Refreshing and Invigorating Baths

| | | | | | | |
|---|---|---|---|---|---|---|
| juniper | 3 | juniper | 3 | juniper | | 3 |
| mandarin | 3 | tea tree | 3 | lemon | | 3 |
| pine | 2 | grapefruit | 2 | chamomile (M) | | 2 |
| | | | | | | |
| lavender | 4 | lavender | 4 | lavender | | 3 |
| petitgrain | 2 | geranium | 2 | geranium | | 2 |
| orange | 2 | orange | 2 | lemongrass | | 2 |
| | | | | | | |
| rosemary | 3 | geranium | 3 | geranium | | 3 |
| bergamot | 3 | bergamot | 3 | lemon | | 2 |
| lemon | 2 | fennel | 2 | pine | | 2 |
| | | | | | | |
| rosemary | 3 | petitgrain | 3 | mandarin | | 4 |
| juniper | 3 | lime | 2 | bergamot | | 2 |
| eucalyptus | 2 | basil | 2 | peppermint | | 2 |

## Relaxing Evening Baths

| | | | | | | | | |
|---|---|---|---|---|---|---|---|---|
| lavender | 3 | | lavender | 4 | | rosewood | 3 | |
| rose | 3 | | rose | 2 | | lavender | 3 | |
| bergamot | 2 | | ylang-ylang | 2 | | ylang-ylang | 2 | |
| | | | | | | | | |
| lavender | 3 | | lavender | 3 | | sandalwood | 3 | |
| jasmine | 3 | | jasmine | 3 | | rosewood | 3 | |
| lemon | 2 | | sandalwood | 2 | | lavender | 2 | |
| | | | | | | | | |
| sandalwood | 3 | | sandalwood | 3 | | sandalwood | 4 | |
| ylang-ylang | 3 | | ylang-ylang | 3 | | ylang-ylang | 2 | |
| marjoram | 2 | | chamomile (M) | 2 | | geranium | 2 | |
| | | | | | | | | |
| sandalwood | 3 | | sandalwood | 3 | | geranium | 3 | |
| chamomile (M) | 3 | | frankincense | 3 | | frankincense | 3 | |
| geranium | 2 | | geranium | 2 | | cedarwood | 2 | |
| | | | | | | | | |
| rose | 3 | | chamomile (M) | 3 | | rose | 3 | |
| mandarin | 3 | | rose | 3 | | cedarwood | 3 | |
| frankincense | 2 | | cedarwood | 2 | | ylang-ylang | 2 | |
| | | | | | | | | |
| rose | 4 | | jasmine | 3 | | frankincense | 3 | |
| neroli | 2 | | neroli | 3 | | neroli | 3 | |
| mandarin | 2 | | patchouli | 2 | | clary sage | 2 | |
| | | | | | | | | |
| rose | 4 | | orange | 2 | | chamomile (M) | 3 | |
| geranium | 2 | | geranium | 2 | | lavender | 3 | |
| vetivert | 2 | | patchouli | 2 | | geranium | 2 | |

## Warming Winter Baths

| B pepper | 3 | marjoram | 3 | ginger | 3 |
| orange | 2 | clary sage | 2 | sandalwood | 2 |
| lavender | 2 | benzoin | 2 | coriander | 2 |

| marjoram | 3 | cardamon | 3 | B pepper | 3 |
| rosemary | 2 | coriander | 2 | ginger | 2 |
| cardamon | 2 | lavender | 2 | rosemary | 2 |

# ◆ Massage

Add each recipe to 25 ml of vegetable oil.

## *Relaxing Massage*

| | | | | | | *Floral* | | |
|---|---|---|---|---|---|---|---|---|
| lavender | 3 | | frankincense | 3 | | jasmine | 3 | |
| geranium | 2 | | lavender | 3 | ✗ | lavender | 2 | ✗ |
| melissa | 2 | | geranium | 2 | | geranium | 2 | |
| | | | | | | | | |
| neroli | 2 | ✗ | frankincense | 3 | | cedarwood | 3 | |
| geranium | 2 | | geranium | 2 | ✗ | sandalwood | 3 | ✗ |
| rosewood | 2 | | rosewood | 2 | | rosewood | 2 | |
| | | | | | | | | |
| benzoin | 3 | | benzoin | 4 | | benzoin | 4 | |
| rose | 3 | ✗ | rosewood | 2 | ✗ | ylang-ylang | 2 | ✗ |
| marjoram | 2 | | neroli | 2 | | frankincense | 2 | |
| | | | | | | | | |
| chamomile (M) | 3 | | chamomile (M) | 2 | | neroli | 3 | |
| cedarwood | 2 | | rosewood | 2 | | chamomile (M) | 2 | |
| ylang-ylang | 2 | | mandarin | 2 | | lavender | 2 | |
| | | | | | | | | |
| clary sage | 3 | | nutmeg | 3 | | mandarin | 3 | |
| mandarin | 2 | ✗ | mandarin | 2 | | lavender | 2 | ✗ |
| geranium | 2 | | geranium | 2 | | ylang-ylang | 2 | |

*Aromatherapy Blends and Remedies*

| | | | | | | | |
|---|---|---|---|---|---|---|---|
| frankincense | 3 | vetivert | 2 | lemon | 3 | |
| bergamot | 2 | bergamot | 2 | vetivert | 2 | |
| cedarwood | 2 | rosewood | 2 | jasmine | 2 | |

| | | | | | | | |
|---|---|---|---|---|---|---|---|
| benzoin | 3 | neroli | 3 | marjoram | 3 | |
| bergamot | 3 | bergamot | 2 | geranium | 2 | |
| clary sage | 2 | patchouli | 2 | patchouli | 2 | |

## Uplifting Massage

| | | | | | | | |
|---|---|---|---|---|---|---|---|
| juniper | 4 | lemongrass | 4 | rosemary | 4 | |
| eucalyptus | 4 | eucalyptus | 3 | eucalyptus | 3 | |
| mandarin | 2 | mandarin | 2 | lemon | 3 | |

| | | | | | | | |
|---|---|---|---|---|---|---|---|
| rosemary | 5 | rosemary | 5 | rosemary | 4 | |
| geranium | 3 | geranium | 3 | bergamot | 3 | |
| peppermint | 2 | lime | 3 | lemon | 3 | |

| | | | | | | |
|---|---|---|---|---|---|---|
| grapefruit | 4 | petitgrain | 4 | bergamot | 4 |
| coriander | 3 | coriander | 3 | coriander | 4 |
| B pepper | 3 | grapefruit | 3 | geranium | 2 |

| | | | | | | | |
|---|---|---|---|---|---|---|---|
| petitgrain | 4 | petitgrain | 4 | pine | 4 | |
| orange | 3 | lemon | 3 | petitgrain | 3 | |
| bergamot | 2 | B pepper | 3 | lemon | 3 | |

| | | | | | | |
|---|---|---|---|---|---|---|
| juniper | 5 | juniper | 4 | basil | 5 |
| orange | 3 | lemon | 3 | juniper | 3 |
| lime | 3 | geranium | 2 | grapefruit | 2 |

| | | | | | | |
|---|---|---|---|---|---|---|
| palmarosa | 4 | niaouli | 4 | fennel | 4 |
| juniper | 3 | palmarosa | 3 | palmarosa | 3 |
| pine | 3 | lemon | 3 | bergamot | 3 |

| | | | | | | | | |
|---|---|---|---|---|---|---|---|---|
| juniper | 4 | | fennel | 4 | | mandarin | | |
| melissa | 3 | | lime | 3 | | nutmeg | 4 | |
| petitgrain | 3 | | cypress | 3 | | anise | 2 | |

## Sensual Massage

| | | | | | | | | |
|---|---|---|---|---|---|---|---|---|
| sandalwood | 5 | | sandalwood | 5 | | sandalwood | 5 | |
| jasmine | 4 | | jasmine | 4 | | rose | 4 | |
| ylang-ylang | 4 | | rose | 3 | | clary sage | 3 | |
| | | | | | | | | |
| ylang-ylang | 4 | | jasmine | 4 | | jasmine | 4 | |
| neroli | 4 | | cedarwood | 4 | | rose | 4 | |
| clary sage | 4 | | clary sage | 3 | | clary sage | 3 | |
| | | | | | | | | |
| frankincense | 5 | | frankincense | 5 | | nutmeg | 5 | |
| neroli | 4 | | cedarwood | 4 | | frankincense | 4 | |
| vetivert | 3 | | jasmine | 3 | | jasmine | 4 | |
| | | | | | | | | |
| ylang-ylang | 5 | | rose | 4 | | rose | 5 | |
| neroli | 3 | | neroli | 4 | | sandalwood | 4 | |
| vetivert | 3 | | vetivert | 4 | | vetivert | 3 | |
| | | | | | | | | |
| nutmeg | 5 | | nutmeg | 4 | | nutmeg | 5 | |
| cedarwood | 5 | | ylang-ylang | 4 | | neroli | 4 | |
| rose | 3 | | rose | 3 | | jasmine | 3 | |
| | | | | | | | | |
| jasmine | 4 | | patchouli | 4 | | frankincense | 5 | |
| patchouli | 4 | | neroli | 4 | | neroli | 4 | |
| neroli | 3 | | sandalwood | 3 | | rose | 3 | |

# ◆ Face and Bodycare

## Face Care

### Abscesses and Boils

|  | Compress | Cream |
|---|---|---|
| bergamot | 1 drop | 5 drops |
| chamomile (R) | 1 drop | 4 drops |
| tea tree | 1 drop | 3 drops |

First apply a hot compress of 1 drop of each oil listed above.

Then add the number of drops listed above in the second column to a 30-g jar of cream and apply directly to the area to be treated.

### Blackheads and Spots

| | |
|---|---|
| pine | 2 drops |
| eucalyptus | 2 drops |
| lavender | 2 drops |

First use the steaming method with the above oils, which is also good for cleansing congested skin.

Then mix the oils listed below with a little jojoba oil, add to a 30-g jar of cream and apply to the area to be treated.

| lemon | 3 drops |
|---|---|
| lavender | 4 drops |

*Scars*

| lavender | 4 drops |
|---|---|
| neroli | 2 drops |
| wheatgerm | 15 drops |

Add to a 30-g jar of cream or, alternatively, blend with 10 ml of jojoba oil and apply to the area to be treated.

For the following recipes, add the essential oils to 10 ml of jojoba oil and apply to the area to be treated.

*Melanosis (dark pigmentation) and Freckles (to lighten)*

| neroli | 2 drops |
|---|---|
| lemon | 1 drop |
| chamomile (R) | 3 drops |

*Broken Capillaries or Thread Veins*

| neroli | 2 drops |
|---|---|
| chamomile (R) | 3 drops |
| rose | 1 drop |

*Blemishes*

| carrot seed | 2 drops |
|---|---|
| chamomile (R) | 3 drops |

### Eczema (patchy, dry, itchy skin)

chamomile (R)     2 drops
evening primrose  10 drops

### Acne

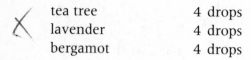

tea tree   4 drops
lavender   4 drops
bergamot   4 drops

The following recipes are for treating different skin types:

### Sensitive Skin

chamomile (R)  1 drop
rose           1 drop
lavender       1 drop

Add to a 30-g jar of cream or blend with 10 ml of jojoba oil.

### Oily Skin

bergamot   2 drops
cedarwood  2 drops
geranium   1 drop

Add to 10 ml of jojoba oil.

### Dry Skin

sandalwood  3 drops
rose        2 drops
geranium    1 drop

Blend with 5 ml of avocado oil and 5 ml of jojoba oil.

| *Mature Skin* | | *Wrinkles* | |
|---|---|---|---|
| frankincense | 2 drops | carrot seed | 2 drops |
| rose | 1 drop | neroli | 1 drop |
| carrot seed | 2 drops | frankincense | 2 drops |

For each recipe, blend the essential oils with 5 ml of peach kernel oil and 5 ml of jojoba oil.

| *Nourishing Night Cream* | | *Toning Blend* | |
|---|---|---|---|
| rose | 2 drops | lavender | 2 drops |
| jasmine | 2 drops | rose | 1 drop |
| evening primrose | 6 drops | neroli | 2 drops |
| peach kernel | 10 drops | | |

Add to a 30-g jar of cream.     Add to 10 ml of jojoba oil.

## Hair Care

*Head Infestations (Lice or Nits)*

| | |
|---|---|
| eucalyptus | 8 drops |
| tea tree | 10 drops |
| thyme | 7 drops |

Add to 50 ml of jojoba oil. Apply evenly to the hair and scalp. Leave for two hours, then wash thoroughly. Towel dry the hair. Pour half a cup of vodka into an empty bottle, add the above essential oils and shake well. Slowly apply your mix to the scalp, comb through the hair and leave for half an hour. Rinse thoroughly with warm water.

**Precaution:**
Do not let the preparation drip into the eyes.

It is not advisable to leave young children unattended during this treatment, as undoubtedly they will scratch and play with the hair and accidentally touch their eyes.

For children between three and eight years old, use half the amount of each of the essential oils.

### To Stimulate Hair Growth

| | |
|---|---|
| rosemary | 10 drops |
| bay | 8 drops |
| cedarwood | 7 drops |

### Dandruff

| | |
|---|---|
| rosemary | 8 drops |
| cedarwood | 8 drops |
| cypress | 5 drops |

### Psoriasis of the Scalp

| | |
|---|---|
| chamomile (R) | 8 drops |
| evening primrose | 25 drops |

Add the above recipes to 50 ml of jojoba oil. Apply to the scalp, cover with a towel or shower cap and leave overnight. Wash your hair the next morning.

### Conditioner for Dry Hair

| | |
|---|---|
| geranium | 10 drops |
| sandalwood | 15 drops |

### Conditioner for Oily Hair

| | |
|---|---|
| bergamot | 10 drops |
| cedarwood | 15 drops |

Add to 50 ml of jojoba oil. Apply to the hair and scalp. Wrap your hair in a towel and leave for approximately two hours. Wash your hair with a mild shampoo.

| *Tonic for Fair Hair* | | *Tonic for Dark Hair* | |
|---|---|---|---|
| chamomile (R) | 15 drops | rosemary | 15 drops |
| lemon | 10 drops | rosewood | 10 drops |

Add to 50 ml of jojoba oil. Apply to the hair and scalp. Wrap your hair in a towel and leave for approximately two hours. Wash your hair with a mild shampoo.

| *Rinse for Fair Hair* | *Rinse for Dark Hair* |
|---|---|
| chamomile (R) 4 drops | rosewood 4 drops |

To your final rinse, fill a jug with warm water and add your chosen essential oil, stir well and pour through the hair.

| *Mouth Ulcers* | | *Bad Breath and Sore Throat* | |
|---|---|---|---|
| myrrh | 1 drop | eucalyptus | 2 drops |
| tea tree | 1 drop | tea tree | 2 drops |

| | |
|---|---|
| Dab on neat with cotton bud. | For gargle or mouthwash, add to a tumbler of warm water. |

## Hand, Feet and Nail Care

| *Dry Hands* | | *Chapped Hands* | |
|---|---|---|---|
| rose | 3 drops | benzoin | 5 drops |
| sandalwood | 6 drops | myrrh | 3 drops |
| geranium | 2 drops | frankincense | 4 drops |
| evening primrose | 10 drops | evening primrose | 20 drops |

Blend each recipe with 10 ml of avocado oil and 15 ml of jojoba oil.

*Aromatherapy Blends and Remedies*

### Brittle Nails

| | |
|---|---|
| rosemary | 6 drops |
| lemon | 3 drops |
| frankincense | 5 drops |

Blend with 5 ml of wheatgerm oil and 20 ml of almond oil.

### Nail Strengthener

| | |
|---|---|
| rosemary | 6 drops |
| carrot seed | 6 drops |
| evening primrose | 15 drops |

Add to 25 ml of jojoba oil.

Massage each recipe (as needed) into the nail area and around the cuticles.

### Warts, Verrucas and Corns

 lemon or tea tree

### Whitlow and Nail-bed Infection

tea tree or thyme

For each condition, apply neat essential oil directly to the area. Try to avoid the healthy surrounding skin.

### Sweaty Feet

| | |
|---|---|
| cypress | 6 drops |
| tea tree | 3 drops |

Add to a bowl of warm water and soak the feet.

### Athlete's Foot

Apply tea tree neat.

### Foot Cramps

| | |
|---|---|
| rosemary | 6 drops |
| B pepper | 6 drops |

Add to 25 ml of vegetable oil. Gently massage the foot and toes.

### Chilblains

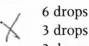

| | |
|---|---|
| rosemary | 6 drops |
| peppermint | 3 drops |
| lavender | 3 drops |

Add to a bowl of tepid water and soak the feet. Then blend the above oils, add to a 30-g jar of cream and apply to the toes.

# ◆ First-Aid and Holidays

Unless otherwise indicated, the following blends should be mixed into a 30-g jar of fragrance- and lanolin-free cream.

## Mosquito Repellent

citronella        15 drops

Use sparingly on the neck, arms and legs. Also add to a handkerchief or a burner. (Do not use vegetable oils for a base as this will attract insects.)

## Bites and Stings

Dab a little neat lavender directly onto the bite or sting. This will ease the discomfort and aid the healing process.

## Minor Cuts and Grazes

| | |
|---|---|
| tea tree | 6 drops |
| lemon | 4 drops |
| thyme | 4 drops |

## Cold Sores

| | |
|---|---|
| lavender | 6 drops |
| eucalyptus | 4 drops |
| tea tree | 4 drops |

## Heat Rash

| | |
|---|---|
| lavender | 6 drops |
| chamomile (R) | 6 drops |

## Head Clearing

| | |
|---|---|
| lavender | 6 drops |
| peppermint | 4 drops |

*Aromatherapy Blends and Remedies*

*Sunburn*

lavender       8 drops
peppermint     4 drops

Alternatively, add the
same amount of drops
to a tablespoon of jojoba
oil and soak in a cool bath
for 10 minutes.

*Chapped Lips*

benzoin        8 drops
lavender       4 drops

Add to 25 ml of avocado
oil.

The following blends are for mixing in water.

*Cuts and Grazes*

tea tree       6 drops

Add to 500 ml water and bathe the affected area.

*Aching Feet*

peppermint     6 drops
rosemary       3 drops

Add to a bowl of cool water and soak the feet for approximately
10 minutes.

Add the following blends to 50 ml of vegetable oil.

### Puffy Legs and Ankles

| | |
|---|---|
| rosemary | 10 drops |
| juniper | 9 drops |
| fennel | 6 drops |

Massage in circular, upward movements.

### Constipation

| | |
|---|---|
| rosemary | 10 drops |
| marjoram | 9 drops |
| B pepper | 6 drops |

Massage over abdomen and lower back.

### Muscle Strain

| | |
|---|---|
| lavender | 10 drops |
| B pepper | 9 drops |
| lemongrass | 6 drops |

### After-sun Oil

| | |
|---|---|
| geranium | 10 drops |
| lavender | 9 drops |
| chamomile (R) | 6 drops |

## Sunbathing

Whilst sunbathing, avocado oil will help to protect your skin from dehydration, at the same time giving you a beautiful golden tan. (Always remember to use a sun-screen on the most sensitive parts of your body.)

### Dry or Damaged Hair

Apply jojoba oil to the hair and scalp. For best results leave on while sunbathing. (It is sufficient on its own; you do not need to add any essential oils.)

### Dehydrated and Dry Skin

• For the Body – Add 15 drops of geranium in 50 ml of avocado oil.

- For the Face – Add 3 drops of neroli in 10 ml of jojoba oil.

## Bruising

cypress       10 drops
hyssop         5 drops

## Travel Sickness

Dab a few drops of ginger and peppermint to a paper tissue or handkerchief and inhale.

## Toothache

Apply 1 or 2 drops of clove oil directly to the cavity in the tooth. (Try to avoid the tongue.)

# ◆ Pregnancy, Mother and Baby

In pregnancy, aromatherapy helps to relieve many problems such as morning sickness, varicose veins, oedema, backache and stretch marks. It will also help to minimize labour pains, re-tone the mother's body after giving birth, and balance the moods.

## Adverse Publicity

Nowadays there is a lot of talk of the 'dangers' of aromatherapy. It is unfortunate that what is written on the toxicity of using essential oils during pregnancy is out of context and greatly exaggerated, and that long lists of essential oils have been prohibited without any explanation or reasoning for the ban.

Many pregnant women were using essential oils rationally at the usual 2–5 per cent dilution in aromatherapy for a long time without any adverse effects before the recent panic about the dangers of aromatherapy in pregnancy. It is not uncommon for many women to be unaware that they are pregnant until several weeks (3 to 6) into their pregnancy. They therefore do not make any changes to their normal daily conduct, including perhaps having aromatherapy treatments. None has shown any adverse reactions as a result of these treatments.

It is certainly sensible to be aware of the potential hazards of inappropriate use, misuse or abuse, especially of some of the more powerful essential oils, but projecting irrational fears and frightening the public is both unreasonable and unnecessary.

Some essential oils, such as pennyroyal, sage and thuja, have acquired a notorious reputation for being dangerous in pregnancy. This is because some desperate women have ingested large quantities (30 ml of the pure essential oil) to bring on miscarriage, and have harmed themselves in doing so.

The public should be warned instead that there are publicity-seeking articles quoting lists of 'DANGEROUS OILS TO BE AVOIDED AT ALL COSTS'. This sort of language simply shows the paranoia of the writers. Some of these comments are written by journalists who have obviously not done any research; others, unfortunately, are written by so-called aromatherapists with very poor training and little knowledge of their subject.

Among the more responsible aromatherapists, it is clear that the real problem in aromatherapy is actually the improper use of essential oils.

## Aromatherapy Massage

Although pregnancy is often quoted as a contra-indication for massage, this is not the case. Massage is actually beneficial during the entire nine-month period of pregnancy. Massage is especially useful in preparing the mother's body for the birth (and is often also beneficial to the baby).

During pregnancy, massage can be carried out on any part of the body, but light pressure is recommended. However, during the first three months of pregnancy it is best to avoid the lower abdomen. Usually most women will experience some discomfort lying face down from the fourth or fifth month onwards. Massage should then be carried out with the mother lying on her side.

An alternative and often preferable position is for the mother to sit on a stool facing the back of an armchair or couch and resting her folded forearms on the seatback or couch in front of her. Another alternative for back and shoulder massage is to sit astride a chair facing the back, supported by cushions. Do not massage if the mother feels nauseated or unwell. Always seek medical advice if unsure of a problem or if complications arise.

Aromatic baths are also very beneficial to the expectant mother throughout pregnancy. During and after pregnancy the skin can be very sensitive. It is advisable to add your essential oils to a teaspoon of jojoba oil before adding them to the bath water.

## Safe Treatments

An important consideration in the safety of aromatherapy treatments during pregnancy is the obstetrical history of the mother. More restrictive use of essential oils should be considered for women with previous miscarriages or those in other high-risk categories. Always seek medical advice if unsure. If used in large quantities, some essential oils can be emmenagogic, such as angelica, carrot, cumin, juniper, parsley, and sage. However, when used in a 1 per cent blend for massage, even these do not pose a problem.

*Relaxing Massage Blends*

| neroli | 4 | neroli | 4 | neroli | 4 |
| lavender | 3 | sandalwood | 4 | clary sage | 3 |

| rose | 5 | rose | 4 | rose | 4 |
| chamomile (R) | 3 | frankincense | 4 | ylang-ylang | 3 |

*Blends for Minor Problems During Pregnancy*

For massage, add each recipe to 25 ml of vegetable oil.

*Fatigue*

| lavender | 5 |
| bergamot | 5 |

*Fluid Retention*

| rosemary | 6 |
| geranium | 4 |

201

*Aromatherapy Blends and Remedies*

| | | | | | |
|---|---|---|---|---|---|
| **Indigestion/Heartburn** | | | **Insomnia** | | |
| lemon | 6 | | sandalwood | 6 | |
| peppermint | 4 | | lavender | 4 | |

*Indigestion/Heartburn*

lemon    6
peppermint    4

*Insomnia*

sandalwood    6
lavender    4

*Leg Cramps*

rosemary    6
chamomile (R)    4

*Mood Swings*

bergamot    6
geranium    4

*Nausea (a recipe for inhalation)*

peppermint    3
ginger    3

*Sore Breasts*

geranium    5
lavender    5

*Stretch Marks*

lavender    5
mandarin    5

*Varicose Veins*

cypress    6
geranium    4

*Essential Oils for Labour*

*For Room Vaporization*

Essential oils can be burned in the room to provide a joyful atmosphere. The number of drops do not have to be exact. The following blends are especially good:

- geranium, lemon and neroli
- geranium, lemon and juniper
- frankincense, lemon and mandarin
- lavender, peppermint and mandarin    Vaporiser.
- bergamot, grapefruit and cedarwood

202

## Massage Blends during Labour

For massage add each recipe to 25 ml of vegetable oil.

Gentle massage with essential oils is of enormous help during this time of apprehension and anxiety, and will help the mother to relax.

| | | | | | | | |
|---|---|---|---|---|---|---|---|
| neroli | 4 | neroli | 4 | jasmine | 4 | rose | 5 |
| jasmine | 3 | geranium | 3 | marjoram | 3 | lavender | 3 |

## Looking after Yourself after Baby's Birth

It is important to continue caring for yourself after the birth. The following are some common problems that may occur and the essential oils that will be helpful. Add each recipe to 25 ml of vegetable oil, unless the recipe states otherwise.

### Aching Legs

| | |
|---|---|
| rosemary | 5 |
| marjoram | 4 |
| lavender | 3 |

### Cellulite

| | |
|---|---|
| juniper | 5 |
| rosemary | 4 |
| geranium | 3 |

### Re-toning

| | |
|---|---|
| rosemary | 4 |
| lemon | 4 |
| B pepper | 4 |

### Sore Nipples

| | |
|---|---|
| benzoin | 4 |
| rose | 3 |
| chamomile (R) | 2 |

### Mastitis

| | |
|---|---|
| rose | 4 |
| geranium | 4 |
| chamomile (R) | 3 |

### Weak Immunity

| | |
|---|---|
| tea tree | 5 |
| bergamot | 4 |
| niaouli | 3 |

## Vaginal Pruritus

| | |
|---|---|
| chamomile (R) | 4 |
| bergamot | 3 |
| tea tree | 3 |

Add to 30 g of cream.

## Thrush

| | |
|---|---|
| myrrh | 4 |
| cinnamon | 3 |

Add to 30 g of cream.

## Invigorating Blends

### For Room Vaporization

bergamot, rosemary and grapefruit
juniper, eucalyptus and lemon
petitgrain, neroli and orange
basil, mandarin and juniper

## Invigorating and Refreshing Blends

If using these blends for massage, add each recipe to 25 ml of vegetable oil.

For baths, use half the number of drops indicated for each recipe.

| | | | |
|---|---|---|---|
| bergamot | 4 | juniper | 4 |
| rosemary | 3 | grapefruit | 4 |
| eucalyptus | 3 | geranium | 2 |
| | | | |
| lemon | 4 | lemon | 4 |
| rosemary | 3 | juniper | 3 |
| lime | 2 | pine | 3 |

## Baby Massage

Gentle massage with essential oils will help to calm and relax your baby. When massaging the baby, use only a small amount of your massage blend, avoiding baby's face and hands, as this poses the risk of passing the oil to the mouth or eyes.

Always use upward strokes and circular movements in a rhythmic flow. Before lifting baby, remember to dab off any excess oil from his body and to wipe your own hands, as your baby may be left quite oily and may slip out of your hands.

## *Relaxing Blends for Baby Massage*

Add one drop of each essential oil from any of the following six recipes to 10 ml of jojoba oil.

| | |
|---|---|
| lavender and chamomile (R) | lavender and sandalwood |
| lavender and mandarin | lavender and frankincense |
| lavender and geranium | lavender and rose |

## *Blends for Baby's Minor Problems*

### *Nappy Rash*

| | |
|---|---|
| chamomile (R) | 2 drops |
| lavender | 1 drop |
| evening primrose | 10 drops |

Add to 30 g of cream.

### *Colic*

| | |
|---|---|
| chamomile (R) | 2 drops |

Add to 10 ml jojoba oil.

Gently massage baby's tummy in a circular, clockwise direction.

*Teething*

| | |
|---|---|
| lavender | 1 drop |
| chamomile (R) | 1 drop |

Add to 30 g cream. Apply to baby's jawline.

*Cradle Cap (flaky patches on the scalp)*

Gently apply a small amount of jojoba oil to the scalp twice daily.

*Eczema*

Add 1 teaspoonful of jojoba oil to baby's bath.

   This will moisturize baby's skin and help to stop itching due to dryness of the skin. (Always seek professional advice if the condition worsens.)

*Stuffy Cold*

benzoin and niaouli or eucalyptus and lemon   ✓

Add the essential oils to your essential oil burner to help baby breathe easier; at the same time these oils will kill any airborne bacteria.

*Baby's Bath Time*

For a baby's bath, use only 1–2 drops of essential oils. If you do not wish to dilute your essential oils in jojoba oil first, be especially careful as babies and young children love to splash and play in the bath and can easily get essential oils on their hands – if these are then rubbed into the eyes or placed in the mouth, they can cause much discomfort and lead to more serious skin irritation problems.

# ◆ For Men

Most men seem to dislike being massaged with sweet, flowery blends. The following blends are specially formulated for their preference. They are particularly suited to either massage or use in essential oil burners.

Blends for massage: add each recipe to 25 ml of vegetable oil.

For room vaporization: use the same number of drops as indicated below.

## Relaxing Blends

| | | | | |
|---|---|---|---|---|
| frankincense | 5 | sandalwood | 5 | |
| orange | 4 | orange | 4 | |
| myrrh | 2 | vetivert | 2 | |
| | | | | |
| lemon | 5 | lemon | 3 | |
| patchouli | 5 | benzoin | 3 | |
| frankincense | 2 | cedarwood | 2 | |
| | | | | |
| grapefruit | 4 | mandarin | 4 | |
| frankincense | 3 | cedarwood | 3 | |
| cedarwood | 3 | vetivert | 2 | |
| | | | | |
| juniper | 3 | palmarosa | 5 | |
| sandalwood | 2 | sandalwood | 3 | |
| myrrh | 2 | patchouli | 3 | |

207

## Aromatherapy Blends and Remedies

| | | | | | |
|---|---|---|---|---|---|
| patchouli | 3 | | orange | 4 | |
| bergamot | 2 | | lavender | 2 | |
| lemon | 2 | | marjoram | 2 | |
| | | | | | |
| bergamot | 3 | | sandalwood | 3 | |
| ginger | 2 | | ginger | 2 | |
| clary sage | 2 | | lavender | 2 | |

## Invigorating Blends

| | | | | |
|---|---|---|---|---|
| grapefruit | 3 | coriander | 3 |
| lemon | 3 | lime | 3 |
| melissa | 2 | mandarin | 2 |
| | | | |
| B pepper | 4 | coriander | 3 |
| orange | 2 | bergamot | 3 |
| juniper | 2 | juniper | 2 |
| | | | |
| B pepper | 3 | cinnamon | 2 |
| rosemary | 3 | rosemary | 2 |
| lemongrass | 2 | petitgrain | 2 |
| | | | |
| petitgrain | 4 | cypress | 3 |
| lemon | 3 | lime | 3 |
| basil | 2 | petitgrain | 2 |
| | | | |
| pine | 2 | cypress | 3 |
| bergamot | 2 | bergamot | 2 |
| grapefruit | 2 | orange | 2 |
| | | | |
| lemon | 4 | lemon | 3 |
| rosemary | 2 | eucalyptus | 3 |
| pine | 2 | juniper | 3 |

| rosemary | 2 | mandarin | 4 |
| lavender | 2 | thyme | 3 |
| basil | 2 | cypress | 2 |

| grapefruit | 3 | petitgrain | 3 |
| palmarosa | 2 | pine | 2 |
| niaouli | 2 | lavender | 2 |

# ◆ Digestive Disorders

For massage, add each recipe to 25 ml of vegetable oil.

| *Anorexia* | | *Appetite, Loss of* | |
|---|---|---|---|
| bergamot | 6 | bergamot | 5 |
| angelica | 2 | B pepper | 4 |
| cardamon | 2 | coriander | 2 |
| or | | or | |
| lime | 4 | lemon | 6 |
| nutmeg | 4 | angelica | 3 |
| coriander | 2 | thyme | 2 |

| *Constipation* | | *Cramps* | |
|---|---|---|---|
| rosemary | 5 | rosemary | 6 |
| B pepper | 4 | fennel | 4 |
| orange | 4 | peppermint | 2 |
| or | | or | |
| B pepper | 5 | marjoram | 5 |
| basil | 4 | anise | 4 |
| neroli | 2 | melissa | 2 |

## Flatulent Colic

| | | | |
|---|---|---|---|
| mandarin | 5 | marjoram | 5 |
| nutmeg | 4 | basil | 3 |
| peppermint | 2 | cardamon | 2 |

or

or

| | | | |
|---|---|---|---|
| juniper | 4 | juniper | 4 |
| anise | 3 | B pepper | 3 |
| melissa | 2 | rosemary | 3 |

## Heartburn

## Hiccups

| | | | |
|---|---|---|---|
| marjoram | 5 | mandarin | 5 |
| chamomile (R) | 4 | basil | 4 |
| peppermint | 2 | cardamon | 2 |

## Indigestion

| | | | |
|---|---|---|---|
| lemon | 4 | lime | 5 |
| anise | 3 | anise | 4 |
| B pepper | 3 | chamomile (R) | 3 |

or

or

| | | | |
|---|---|---|---|
| orange | 5 | orange | 5 |
| marjoram | 4 | fennel | 4 |
| clove | 3 | sage | 3 |

or

or

| | | | |
|---|---|---|---|
| mandarin | 6 | lime | 4 |
| cinnamon | 4 | rosemary | 4 |
| peppermint | 2 | nutmeg | 3 |

| or | | or | |
|---|---|---|---|
| grapefruit | 5 | juniper | 5 |
| ginger | 4 | cardamon | 3 |
| coriander | 3 | basil | 2 |

| *Jaundice* | | *Vomiting* | |
|---|---|---|---|
| juniper | 5 | basil | 4 |
| grapefruit | 4 | chamomile (R) | 2 |
| rosemary | 3 | cinnamon | 2 |

| or | | or | |
|---|---|---|---|
| lemon | 5 | ginger | 3 |
| fennel | 3 | nutmeg | 2 |
| chamomile (R) | 3 | peppermint | 2 |

# ◆ Urinary Disorders

For massage, add each recipe to 25 ml of vegetable oil. For baths, use half the amount of drops indicated for each recipe.

| *Cystitis* | | *Oedema* | |
|---|---|---|---|
| tea tree | 5 | celery | 5 |
| lavender | 4 | rosemary | 5 |
| bergamot | 3 | grapefruit | 3 |
| or | | or | |
| cedarwood | 6 | fennel | 5 |
| geranium | 4 | geranium | 4 |
| carrot | 2 | parsley | 3 |
| or | | or | |
| sandalwood | 5 | rosemary | 5 |
| celery | 4 | juniper | 5 |
| chamomile (R) | 3 | celery | 3 |
| or | | or | |
| juniper | 5 | fennel | 5 |
| benzoin | 5 | juniper | 5 |
| rosemary | 2 | parsley | 3 |

| *Toxic Accumulation* | | | *Urine Retention* | |
|---|---|---|---|---|
| celery | 5 | | B pepper | 4 |
| grapefruit | 4 | | anise | 4 |
| fennel | 3 | | rosemary | 4 |
| or | | | or | |
| rosemary | 5 | | juniper | 5 |
| juniper | 5 | | fennel | 5 |
| celery | 3 | | cardamon | 2 |
| or | | | or | |
| rosemary | 5 | | celery | 5 |
| fennel | 5 | | fennel | 5 |
| carrot seed | 3 | | carrot | 3 |

# ◆ Circulatory Disorders

For massage, add each recipe to 25 ml of vegetable oil.

| *Anaemia* | | | *Blood Pressure, High* | |
|---|---|---|---|---|
| rose | 4 | | rose | 4 |
| B pepper | 4 | | celery | 3 |
| angelica | 2 | | neroli | 3 |
| or | | | or | |
| rose | 6 | | ylang-ylang | 5 |
| angelica | 2 | | lavender | 4 |
| sage | 2 | | clary sage | 3 |

| *Blood Pressure, Low* | | | *Circulation, Poor* | |
|---|---|---|---|---|
| B pepper | 5 | | rosemary | 4 |
| rosemary | 4 | | angelica | 4 |
| camphor | 3 | | ginger | 3 |
| or | | | or | |
| rosemary | 6 | | rose | 4 |
| camphor | 3 | | B pepper | 4 |
| thyme | 3 | | thyme | 2 |

## Haemorrhoids

| | |
|---|---|
| cypress | 4 |
| lemon | 4 |
| chamomile (R) | 3 |

## Heart, Weak

| | |
|---|---|
| rosemary | 5 |
| rose | 4 |
| angelica | 2 |

or

| | |
|---|---|
| ylang-ylang | 5 |
| hyssop | 3 |
| melissa | 2 |

or

| | |
|---|---|
| neroli | 5 |
| rosemary | 4 |
| melissa | 2 |

## Thread Veins

| | |
|---|---|
| neroli | 5 |
| lavender | 3 |
| chamomile (R) | 3 |

## Palpitations

| | |
|---|---|
| lavender | 5 |
| melissa | 4 |
| hyssop | 3 |

or

| | |
|---|---|
| ylang-ylang | 5 |
| neroli | 4 |
| melissa | 2 |

or

| | |
|---|---|
| rose | 4 |
| frankincense | 4 |
| orange | 3 |

or

| | |
|---|---|
| neroli | 5 |
| rose | 4 |
| lavender | 3 |

## Varicose Veins

| | |
|---|---|
| lemon | 5 |
| cypress | 5 |
| geranium | 3 |

# ◆ Respiratory Disorders

The following recipes are for chest rubs. Add each recipe to 25 ml of vegetable oil.

| *Asthma* | | *Bronchitis* | |
|---|---|---|---|
| benzoin | 5 | sandalwood | 6 |
| cypress | 4 | cypress | 5 |
| lavender | 4 | marjoram | 4 |
| or | | or | |
| frankincense | 5 | cedarwood | 6 |
| benzoin | 5 | hyssop | 4 |
| chamomile (R) | 3 | pine | 3 |
| or | | or | |
| frankincense | 5 | ginger | 5 |
| benzoin | 5 | niaouli | 4 |
| cypress | 3 | myrrh | 4 |
| or | | or | |
| lavender | 4 | eucalyptus | 5 |
| ylang-ylang | 4 | rosemary | 4 |
| cypress | 4 | pine | 4 |

*Aromatherapy Blends and Remedies*

## Catarrh

| | |
|---|---|
| eucalyptus | 5 |
| marjoram | 4 |
| myrrh | 3 |

or

| | |
|---|---|
| eucalyptus | 5 |
| hyssop | 4 |
| tea tree | 3 |

## Coughs (Dry)

| | |
|---|---|
| sandalwood | 6 |
| anise | 4 |
| peppermint | 2 |

## Coughs (General)

| | |
|---|---|
| rosemary | 4 |
| sage | 4 |
| peppermint | 2 |

or

| | |
|---|---|
| niaouli | 5 |
| hyssop | 4 |
| myrrh | 3 |

## Coughs (Ticklish)

| | |
|---|---|
| marjoram | 5 |
| eucalyptus | 4 |
| lemon | 4 |

## Coughs (Spasmodic)

| | |
|---|---|
| ginger | 5 |
| eucalyptus | 5 |
| cardamon | 3 |

or

| | |
|---|---|
| basil | 5 |
| cypress | 4 |
| tea tree | 3 |

## Coughs (Whooping)

| | |
|---|---|
| lavender | 5 |
| anise | 3 |
| basil | 2 |

or

| | |
|---|---|
| eucalyptus | 4 |
| hyssop | 4 |
| myrrh | 4 |

## Colds

| | |
|---|---|
| lime | 5 |
| cinnamon | 4 |
| peppermint | 2 |

or

| | |
|---|---|
| lemon | 6 |
| clove | 4 |
| myrrh | 3 |

## Flu

| | |
|---|---|
| ginger | 6 |
| rosemary | 5 |
| peppermint | 2 |

or

| | |
|---|---|
| nutmeg | 5 |
| cajeput | 4 |
| rosemary | 3 |

## Emphysema

| | |
|---|---|
| eucalyptus | 5 |
| basil | 4 |
| cypress | 3 |

## Hay Fever

| | |
|---|---|
| pine | 6 |
| eucalyptus | 4 |
| citronella | 4 |

## Laryngitis

| | |
|---|---|
| niaouli | 5 |
| sandalwood | 5 |
| lemongrass | 3 |

## Pleurisy

| | |
|---|---|
| cypress | 4 |
| angelica | 3 |
| cinnamon | 3 |

## Sinusitis

| | |
|---|---|
| pine | 5 |
| eucalyptus | 4 |
| B pepper | 3 |

## Sore Throat

| | |
|---|---|
| pine | 5 |
| benzoin | 5 |
| peppermint | 2 |

| | | | |
|---|---|---|---|
| or | | or | |
| cajeput | 6 | tea tree | 4 |
| cedarwood | 4 | myrrh | 4 |
| basil | 3 | lavender | 4 |

The following recipes are for <u>inhalation</u>.

Add 2 drops of each essential oil indicated for each recipe. For room vaporization, extra drops may be added.

| *Asthma* | *Bronchitis* |
|---|---|
| cypress | benzoin |
| frankincense | hyssop |
| lavender | lavender |
| | |
| or | or |
| | |
| benzoin | thyme |
| marjoram | lemon |
| frankincense | cajeput |

| *Catarrh* | *Coughs* |
|---|---|
| benzoin | benzoin |
| ginger | cardamon |
| pine | marjoram |
| | |
| or | or |
| | |
| hyssop | anise |
| myrrh | juniper |
| lemon | sandalwood |

## Colds

B pepper
camphor
pine

or

thyme
niaouli
marjoram

or

ginger
cinnamon
lemon

## Flu

lavender
eucalyptus
pine

or

pine
lemon
benzoin

or

bay
niaouli
lemon

## Laryngitis

benzoin
lavender
lemongrass

## Pleurisy

niaouli
lavender
pine

## Sinusitis

pine
niaouli
tea tree

or

pine
cajeput
rosemary

## Sore Throat

sandalwood
lavender
benzoin

or

sandalwood
eucalyptus
thyme

# ◆ Reproductive Disorders

For massage, add each recipe to 25 ml of vegetable oil.

| *Infertility* | | | *Leucorrhoea* | |
|---|---|---|---|---|
| rose | 5 | | sandalwood | 5 |
| ylang-ylang | 4 | | rose | 4 |
| clary sage | 3 | | marjoram | 3 |
| or | | | or | |
| rose | 5 | | benzoin | 6 |
| sandalwood | 4 | | bergamot | 4 |
| jasmine | 3 | | lavender | 2 |

| *Menopause* | | | *Premenstrual Cramps* | |
|---|---|---|---|---|
| cypress | 4 | | clary sage | 4 |
| chamomile (R) | 3 | | jasmine | 4 |
| clary sage | 3 | | lavender | 3 |
| or | | | or | |
| geranium | 5 | | cypress | 4 |
| sage | 4 | | chamomile (R) | 4 |
| fennel | 3 | | geranium | 4 |

*Aromatherapy Blends and Remedies*

## Periods, Heavy

| | |
|---|---|
| rose | 5 |
| cypress | 5 |
| angelica | 2 |

## Periods, Irregular

| | |
|---|---|
| rose | 5 |
| fennel | 4 |
| chamomile (R) | 3 |

## Periods, Painful

| | |
|---|---|
| marjoram | 5 |
| rose | 5 |
| clary sage | 3 |

## Periods, Scanty

| | |
|---|---|
| jasmine | 5 |
| lavender | 4 |
| sage | 3 |

# ◆Nervous Disorders

For massage, add each recipe to 25 ml of vegetable oil. For room vaporization, use the same number of drops indicated for each recipe, but for baths use half the number of drops.

| Debility | | Excitability | |
|---|---|---|---|
| mandarin | 6 | ylang-ylang | 6 |
| hyssop | 3 | chamomile (R) | 3 |
| thyme | 2 | lavender | 3 |
| or | | or | |
| jasmine | 5 | rose | 5 |
| marjoram | 3 | marjoram | 4 |
| clary sage | 3 | melissa | 4 |
| or | | or | |
| neroli | 6 | neroli | 4 |
| rosewood | 3 | rosewood | 3 |
| vetivert | 2 | petitgrain | 3 |

| Headaches | | Jet Lag | |
|---|---|---|---|
| lavender | 4 | grapefruit | 5 |
| eucalyptus | 4 | eucalyptus | 3 |
| peppermint | 3 | rosewood | 3 |

## Aromatherapy Blends and Remedies

### Migraine

| | |
|---|---|
| lavender | 5 |
| basil | 3 |
| peppermint | 3 |

### Neuralgia

| | |
|---|---|
| chamomile (R) | 5 |
| rosemary | 4 |
| peppermint | 2 |

### Tension

| | |
|---|---|
| lavender | 4 |
| ylang-ylang | 4 |
| rosewood | 3 |

### Tremblings

| | |
|---|---|
| bergamot | 5 |
| marjoram | 4 |
| lavender | 3 |

# ◆ Muscular Disorders

For massage, add each recipe to 25 ml of vegetable oil. For baths, use half the number of drops indicated for each recipe.

| *Muscles, Painful* | | *Muscles, Tense* | |
|---|---|---|---|
| camphor | 5 | camphor | 5 |
| coriander | 5 | sage | 5 |
| cajeput | 4 | lemongrass | 3 |
| or | | or | |
| rosemary | 5 | basil | 5 |
| marjoram | 5 | marjoram | 4 |
| cinnamon | 3 | pine | 4 |
| or | | or | |
| eucalyptus | 5 | nutmeg | 5 |
| nutmeg | 4 | rosemary | 4 |
| chamomile (R) | 4 | palmarosa | 3 |
| or | | or | |
| B pepper | 5 | B pepper | 5 |
| lavender | 4 | cajeput | 4 |
| nutmeg | 4 | lemongrass | 3 |

| or | | or | |
|---|---|---|---|
| benzoin | 7 | benzoin | 6 |
| thyme | 3 | pine | 4 |
| chamomile (R) | 3 | cardamon | 3 |

| or | | or | |
|---|---|---|---|
| marjoram | 6 | lavender | 5 |
| ginger | 4 | basil | 4 |
| cinnamon | 3 | camphor | 3 |

## Muscles, Tired

| | | ## Rheumatism | |
|---|---|---|---|
| basil | 4 | benzoin | 5 |
| sage | 4 | nutmeg | 4 |
| rosemary | 4 | rosemary | 3 |

| or | | or | |
|---|---|---|---|
| pine | 5 | lavender | 6 |
| lavender | 4 | marjoram | 3 |
| lemongrass | 4 | cinnamon | 3 |

| or | | or | |
|---|---|---|---|
| B pepper | 5 | B pepper | 6 |
| juniper | 5 | cajeput | 3 |
| coriander | 3 | ginger | 3 |

| or | | or | |
|---|---|---|---|
| sage | 5 | lavender | 5 |
| camphor | 4 | coriander | 4 |
| lemongrass | 3 | chamomile (R) | 4 |

## Spasms

| | |
|---|---|
| marjoram | 5 |
| eucalyptus | 4 |
| basil | 4 |

or

| | |
|---|---|
| chamomile (R) | 5 |
| cinnamon | 4 |
| coriander | 3 |

or

| | |
|---|---|
| eucalyptus | 5 |
| chamomile (R) | 4 |
| sage | 3 |

## Sprains

| | |
|---|---|
| marjoram | 4 |
| cajeput | 4 |
| lavender | 4 |

or

| | |
|---|---|
| rosemary | 5 |
| chamomile (R) | 4 |
| clary sage | 3 |

or

| | |
|---|---|
| benzoin | 6 |
| cajeput | 3 |
| basil | 3 |

# ◆ Skeletal Disorders

For massage, add each recipe to 25 ml of vegetable oil. For compresses, use half the number of drops indicated for each recipe.

| *Arthritis* | | *Gout* | |
|---|---|---|---|
| chamomile (G) | 6 | juniper | 6 |
| eucalyptus | 4 | fennel | 4 |
| rosemary | 4 | lemon | 4 |
| or | | or | |
| juniper | 6 | juniper | 5 |
| celery | 4 | rosemary | 5 |
| chamomile (G) | 3 | celery | 3 |

| *Joints, Inflamed* | | *Joints, Painful* | |
|---|---|---|---|
| chamomile (G) | 6 | chamomile (G) | 5 |
| lavender | 4 | juniper | 5 |
| celery | 3 | rosemary | 3 |
| or | | or | |
| lavender | 7 | B pepper | 5 |
| rosemary | 3 | marjoram | 4 |
| eucalyptus | 3 | chamomile (G) | 4 |

## Toxins in the Joints

| | | | |
|---|---|---|---|
| celery | 5 | rosemary | 5 |
| juniper | 4 | juniper | 5 |
| lemon | 4 | geranium | 3 |
| or | | or | |
| rosemary | 4 | juniper | 6 |
| fennel | 4 | lemon | 4 |
| celery | 4 | chamomile (R) | 3 |

# ◆ Skin Disorders

For topical application, add each recipe to 30 g of fragrance- and lanolin-free cream.

| *Acne* | | *Blemishes* | |
|---|---|---|---|
| chamomile (R) | 5 | chamomile (R) | 4 |
| bergamot | 5 | geranium | 3 |
| pine | 3 | carrot | 3 |
| or | | or | |
| tea tree | 5 | jasmine | 3 |
| juniper | 4 | rose | 3 |
| petitgrain | 3 | neroli | 3 |

| *Boils* | | *Bruises* | |
|---|---|---|---|
| lavender | 5 | hyssop | 5 |
| thyme | 4 | niaouli | 5 |
| pine | 3 | caraway | 2 |
| or | | | |
| bergamot | 6 | | |
| niaouli | 4 | | |
| caraway | 2 | | |

## Burns

| | |
|---|---|
| lavender | 6 |
| chamomile (R) | 4 |
| geranium | 3 |

## Cellulite

| | |
|---|---|
| juniper | 6 |
| fennel | 6 |
| geranium | 4 |

## Chilblains

| | |
|---|---|
| benzoin | 6 |
| peppermint | 5 |
| rosemary | 4 |

## Corns

| | |
|---|---|
| lemon | 6 |
| tea tree | 4 |
| melissa | 4 |

## Dermatitis

| | |
|---|---|
| benzoin | 4 |
| chamomile (R) | 3 |
| lavender | 3 |

## Eczema and Psoriasis

| | |
|---|---|
| chamomile (R) | 4 |
| sandalwood | 3 |
| lavender | 3 |

## Eruptions

| | |
|---|---|
| chamomile (R) | 6 |
| cedarwood | 4 |
| eucalyptus | 3 |

## Fungal Infection

| | |
|---|---|
| tea tree | 6 |
| myrrh | 4 |
| citronella | 3 |

## Herpes (Cold Sores)

| | |
|---|---|
| chamomile (R) | 6 |
| bergamot | 6 |
| eucalyptus | 3 |

## Inflammation

| | |
|---|---|
| chamomile (R) | 6 |
| benzoin | 4 |
| frankincense | 4 |

or

| | |
|---|---|
| myrrh | 6 |
| lavender | 4 |
| jasmine | 3 |

or

| | |
|---|---|
| patchouli | 6 |
| sandalwood | 4 |
| rose | 3 |

## Rashes

| | |
|---|---|
| chamomile (R) | 5 |
| benzoin | 4 |
| sandalwood | 3 |

## Scarring

| | |
|---|---|
| lavender | 6 |
| frankincense | 5 |
| neroli | 3 |

or

| | |
|---|---|
| lavender | 5 |
| chamomile (R) | 5 |
| frankincense | 4 |

## Itching

| | |
|---|---|
| lavender | 6 |
| peppermint | 4 |
| cedarwood | 3 |

or

| | |
|---|---|
| chamomile (R) | 6 |
| sandalwood | 4 |
| benzoin | 4 |

or

| | |
|---|---|
| chamomile (R) | 4 |
| lavender | 4 |
| peppermint | 3 |

## Scabies

| | |
|---|---|
| tea tree | 6 |
| thyme | 4 |
| caraway | 2 |

## Skin, Ageing

| | |
|---|---|
| frankincense | 3 |
| jasmine | 3 |
| mandarin | 2 |

or

| | |
|---|---|
| lavender | 3 |
| neroli | 3 |
| myrrh | 2 |

## Skin, Cracked/Chapped

| | |
|---|---|
| benzoin | 6 |
| myrrh | 6 |
| geranium | 3 |

## Shingles

| | |
|---|---|
| tea tree | 6 |
| bergamot | 4 |
| eucalyptus | 4 |

## Sores

| | |
|---|---|
| benzoin | 6 |
| sandalwood | 4 |
| tea tree | 3 |

## Stretch Marks

| | |
|---|---|
| lavender | 6 |
| neroli | 4 |
| mandarin | 3 |

## Sweaty Feet

| | |
|---|---|
| peppermint | 6 |
| cypress | 4 |
| citronella | 3 |

## Ulcers

| | |
|---|---|
| tea tree | 6 |
| myrrh | 4 |
| eucalyptus | 3 |

## Warts

| | |
|---|---|
| tea tree | 6 |
| lemon | 6 |
| thyme | 3 |

## Wounds

| | |
|---|---|
| benzoin | 6 |
| lime | 4 |
| hyssop | 3 |

or

| | |
|---|---|
| myrrh | 6 |
| lemon | 4 |
| eucalyptus | 2 |

or

| | |
|---|---|
| tea tree | 6 |
| geranium | 3 |
| chamomile (R) | 3 |

Aromatherapy Blends and Remedies

*Wrinkles*

| neroli       | 4 |
|--------------|---|
| carrot       | 3 |
| rose         | 3 |

or

| frankincense | 4 |
|--------------|---|
| jasmine      | 4 |
| vetivert     | 3 |

# ◆ Emotional Problems

For room vaporization, add up to a total of 15 drops of oil for each blend.

Please note that throughout this section 'chamomile' refers to either Roman or Maroc, interchangeably.

## Absent-mindedness

cedarwood
ginger
lemon

## Aggression

cedarwood
eucalyptus
lavender

## Agitation

chamomile
lavender
marjoram

or

myrrh
palmarosa
nutmeg

## Alertness, Lack of

peppermint
pine
B pepper

or

lemon
basil
bay

## Anger

chamomile
cedarwood
petitgrain

or

vetivert
ylang-ylang
clary sage

## Anxiety

clove
cedarwood
sandalwood

or

patchouli
neroli
nutmeg

## Apathy

cajeput
camphor
pine

or

rosemary
tea tree
mandarin

## Apprehension

lavender
ylang-ylang
patchouli

or

frankincense
bergamot
juniper

## Awareness, Lack of

frankincense
lemongrass
myrrh

or

bay
hyssop
fennel

## Betrayal, Sense of

petitgrain
peppermint
rosewood

or

pine
juniper
cedarwood

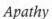

*Bitterness*

lemon
grapefruit
bergamot

or

lime
orange
mandarin

*Clarity, Lack of*

hyssop
cardamon
bergamot

or

palmarosa
peppermint
petitgrain

*Clutter, Emotional*

juniper
sandalwood
clove

or

rose
myrrh
lime

*Clutter, Mental*

juniper
pine
tea tree

or

celery
hyssop
lemon

*Coldness, Emotional*

ginger
marjoram
ylang-ylang

*Compulsiveness*

clary sage
cajeput
patchouli

*Concentration, Poor*

pine
B pepper
rosewood

*Confidence, Lack of*

jasmine
neroli
rose

or

thyme
eucalyptus
petitgrain

or

rosemary
basil
lemon

or

bay
ylang-ylang
bergamot

or

rosemary
rosewood
tea tree

*Conflict*

myrrh
rose
lavender

*Confusion*

cardamon
carrot
niaouli

*Courage, Lack of*

B pepper
thyme
fennel

*Creativity, Lack of*

rosemary
orange
palmarosa

or

frankincense
myrrh
cedarwood

or

basil
grapefruit
coriander

*Crisis*

rose
ylang-ylang
benzoin

*Criticalness, Over-*

jasmine
clary sage
rosewood

## Cynicism

sandalwood
cajeput
bergamot

or

lime
lavender
jasmine

## Daydreaming

cedarwood
camphor
rosewood

or

B pepper
thyme
neroli

## Dejection

melissa
rosewood
juniper

or

orange
peppermint
sandalwood

## Depression

chamomile
benzoin
bergamot

or

grapefruit
geranium
palmarosa

## Despondency

orange
rose
benzoin

## Disorientation

cajeput
rosemary
sandalwood

## Distraction

vetivert
cardamon
rose

## Doubtfulness

carrot
ginger
rose

## Drowsiness

B pepper
nutmeg
patchouli

## Envy

rose
ylang-ylang
jasmine

## Excitement, Over-

carrot
fennel
camphor

## Excitement, Under-

cumin
nutmeg
cedarwood

## Exhaustion, Emotional

benzoin
cinnamon
pine

or

juniper
rosemary
geranium

or

chamomile
marjoram
myrrh

## Fear

vetivert
orange
neroli

or

cedarwood
rosemary
lemon

or

anise
jasmine
ylang-ylang

## Fretfulness

parsley
clary sage
cypress

## Frustration

B pepper
ylang-ylang
grapefruit

## Gloom

orange
rose
benzoin

or

lavender
neroli
clary sage

## Grief

neroli
rose
cypress

or

marjoram
melissa
sage

## Grumpiness

rosewood
lavender
vetivert

## Guilt

rose
sandalwood
ylang-ylang

## Hostility

ylang-ylang
marjoram
clary sage

## Humility

rose
melissa
sandalwood

## Humour, Lack of

lemon
melissa
jasmine

## Hysteria

peppermint
chamomile
clove

## Imagination, Lack of

bay
clary sage
mandarin

## Imaginativeness, Over-

tea tree
lavender
thyme

# Aromatherapy Blends and Remedies

## Impatience

angelica
mandarin
ylang-ylang

## Inability to Meditate

frankincense
myrrh
sandalwood

## Indecisiveness

lavender
lemon
coriander

or

rosemary
grapefruit
angelica

## Indifference

jasmine
patchouli
benzoin

or

juniper
B pepper
angelica

## Inhibitions

jasmine
nutmeg
rosemary

## Insecurity

sandalwood
frankincense
lavender

## Insomnia

lavender
neroli
chamomile

or

bergamot
juniper
marjoram

## Irritability

lavender
marjoram
chamomile

or

ylang-ylang
cypress
sandalwood

## Jealousy

rose
orange
cypress

## Listlessness

palmarosa
coriander
chamomile

## Loneliness

benzoin
cypress
marjoram

## Manic Depression

rose
grapefruit
lavender

## Memory, Poor

caraway
clove
coriander

or

marjoram
peppermint
sage

## Moodiness

bergamot
B pepper
juniper

or

bergamot
geranium
rosewood

## Neglect, Sense of

rosewood
patchouli
orange

## Nervousness

cedarwood
cinnamon
carrot

## Nightmares

thyme
frankincense
lavender

## Obsession

orange
sandalwood
marjoram

Aromatherapy Blends and Remedies

## Paranoia

clary sage
melissa
grapefruit

## Pessimism

jasmine
orange
nutmeg

## Procrastination

sandalwood
grapefruit
cajeput

## Rage

myrrh
neroli
melissa

## Reaction, Over-

myrrh
lavender
clary sage

## Regret

benzoin
rose
bergamot

## Resentment

rose
clary sage
lemon

or

sandalwood
ylang-ylang
geranium

## Restlessness

chamomile
myrrh
melissa

or

sandalwood
jasmine
geranium

## Self-control, Lack of

cedarwood
geranium
lavender

## Selfishness

sandalwood
cardamon
juniper

or

benzoin
bergamot
geranium

or

orange
lemon
ylang-ylang

*Sensitivity, Over-*

chamomile
melissa
vetivert

*Sensitivity, Under-*

rosemary
petitgrain
rose

*Sexual Urge, Strong*

camphor
marjoram
pine

*Sexual Urge, Weak*

rose
jasmine
neroli

or

tea tree
parsley
thyme

or

ylang-ylang
sandalwood
clary sage

*Shock*

neroli
peppermint
benzoin

*Shyness*

ylang-ylang
peppermint
bergamot

*Sluggishness*

rosewood
rosemary
cypress

*Stubbornness*

ylang-ylang
chamomile
orange

*Aromatherapy Blends and Remedies*

### Sulkiness

lemongrass
rosewood
clary sage

### Tantrums

eucalyptus
geranium
chamomile

### Turmoil

lavender
melissa
rosewood

### Weak-willed

pine
petitgrain
B pepper

### Withdrawn

bergamot
ylang-ylang
marjoram

or

basil
geranium
anise

### Worry

juniper
chamomile
lavender

or

frankincense
rosewood
nutmeg

# ◆ Glossary of Medical Terms

| | |
|---|---|
| **Alopecia** | hair loss or baldness |
| **Anaemia** | poor quality of blood |
| **Analgesic** | pain-relieving |
| **Anorexia** | loss of appetite (Anorexia nervosa is the name given to the illness in which the sufferer literally convinces her- or himself that she or he has no appetite) |
| **Anthelmintic** | expels intestinal worms |
| **Anti-emetic** | prevents or stops vomiting |
| **Antihistamine** | counteracts allergic conditions |
| **Anti-inflammatory** | counteracts inflammation |
| **Antiphlogistic** | reduces inflammation |
| **Antispasmodic** | prevents spasms or convulsions |
| **Antiviral** | destroys viruses |
| **Aperitif** | stimulates appetite |
| **Astringent** | contracts or tightens the tissues |
| **Carminative** | relieves flatulence |
| **Cephalic** | head-clearing |
| **Cholagogic** | induces the flow of bile |
| **Cholecystitis** | inflammation of the bile-duct |
| **Choleretic** | promotes the flow of bile |
| **Cicatrizant** | promotes scar formation |
| **Cirrhosis** | degeneration of organ tissue, especially the liver |
| **Colic** | pain due to intestinal cramps |
| **Colitis** | inflammation of the colon |

| | |
|---|---|
| Cordial | stimulant tonic |
| Cystitis | inflammation of the bladder |
| Cytophylactic | promoting cell growth |
| Depurative | blood-cleansing |
| Diuretic | promotes the flow of urine |
| Dysmenorrhoea | painful periods |
| Dyspepsia | indigestion |
| Emmenagogic | promotes menstruation |
| Emollient | softens the skin |
| Emphysema | enlargement of the alveoli in the lungs |
| Euphoric | causing a sense of elation |
| Expectorant | promotes the removal of mucus |
| Fibrositis | inflammation of the connective tissues |
| Gastritis | inflammation of the stomach |
| Gingivitis | inflammation of the gums |
| Gout | inflammation of the joints |
| Haemorrhoids | dilated veins in the anus |
| Haemostatic | arrests bleeding |
| Hepatic | relating to the liver |
| Hepatotoxic | toxic to the liver |
| Hypertensive | raises blood pressure |
| Hypotensive | lowers blood pressure |
| Immunostimulant | stimulates the immune response |
| Jaundice | yellowish colouring of the skin by bile |
| Leucorrhoea | white discharge from the vagina |
| Libido | sexual drive |
| Lipolytic | breaks down fats |
| Mucolytic | breaks down mucus |
| Nausea | unpleasant feeling of vomiting |
| Nervine | soothes nervous excitement |
| Oedema | fluid accumulation beneath the skin |
| Peptic | relating to gastric digestion |
| Peristalsis | wavelike muscular contractions |
| Phototoxic | causing pigmentation and sometimes blistering on exposure to (ultra-violet) light |

| | |
|---|---|
| Pruritus | itching |
| Pulmonary | relating to the lungs |
| Pyelitis | inflammation of the kidneys |
| Rubefacient | causing redness of the skin |
| Seborrhoea | excessive sebum secretion |
| Sedative | reduces functional activity |
| Stimulant | increases functional activity |
| Stomachic | improves appetite |
| Styptic | helps to stop bleeding |
| Sudorific | promotes sweating |
| Tonic | strengthens |
| Urethritis | inflammation of the urine canal from the bladder |
| Urticaria | itching rash |
| Vulnerary | useful in healing wounds |

# ◆ Suggested Reading

Franzesca Watson, *Aromatherapy For You At Home* (Natural by Nature Oils Ltd)

*The MacDonald Encyclopedia of Medicinal Plants* (MacDonald)

Barbara and Peter Theiss, *The Family Herbal* (Healing Arts Press)

Barbara Griggs, *The Green Witch* (Vermilion)

Clare Maxwell-Hudson, *The Complete Book of Massage* (Dorling Kindersley)

C. Beresford-Cooke, *Massage for Healing and Relaxation* (Thames)

Shirley Price, *Aromatherapy Workbook* (Thorsons)

Christine Wildwood, *Creative Aromatherapy* (Thorsons)

Julia Lawless, *Aromatherapy and the Mind* (Thorsons)

Jane Dye, *Aromatherapy for Women and Children* (C. W. Daniel)

Todd and Van Toller, *Perfumery* (Chapman & Hall)Jane Grayson,

The International School of Aromatherapy, *Safety Guide on the Use of Essential Oils* (International School of Aromatherapy)

# ♦ Further Information

## Products and Information

A wide selection of high-quality aromatherapy-grade essential oils, vegetable oils and aromatherapy products is available from:

Natural by Nature Oils Ltd
The Aromatherapy Centre
9 Vivian Avenue
Hendon Central
London NW4 3UT

Tel: 0181–202 5718

An aromatherapy advice line for queries on using essential oils is also available. Please ring the number given above if you wish to find out more, or for your nearest stockist.

## Organizations

Institute of Complementary Medicine
4 Tavern Quay
Plough Way
Surrey Quays
London SE16 1QZ

Tel: 0171–237 5165

The Register of Qualified Aromatherapists
PO Box 6941
London N8 9HF

Tel: 0181–341 2958

American Aromatherapy Association
PO Box 1222
Fair Oaks, CA 95628

## Stockists

Dar-Lin International Esthetic Co.
4th Fl., No. 12, Lane 164
Sung-Chiang Road
Taipei
Taiwan, ROC

Tel: (02) 511 8142

Healthwise (M) Sdn Blvd
51 Jalan SS19/6 Subang Jaya
47500 Petaling Jaya
Selangor
W. Malaysia

Tel: (03) 732 8494

Essensuals
252 Prince's Building
2nd Fl., 10 Chater Road
Hong Kong

Tel: (852) 840 1890

Esthete De Clarte
2–20–8 Shimome Goro
Meguro-Ku
Tokyo
Japan

Tel: (3) 4947610

Rapaura Water Gardens
Tapu Coroglen Road
Tapu PDC
Thames Coast
New Zealand

Paolo Bonnici
Upper Cross Road
Marsa HMR14
Malta

## Treatments

Aromatherapy treatments are available at The Aromatherapy Centre. For appointments telephone 0181–201 5555.

## Training Courses

There are several different courses available, including:

- One- or two-day introductory seminars for beginners who do not wish to train in aromatherapy professionally but would like a basic knowledge of using essential oils safely at home.
- Full diploma training courses for those who seriously wish to practise aromatherapy professionally.

Write with s.a.e. for prospectus of courses and brochures of

255

seminars to:
The International School of Aromatherapy at the address given above for the Aromatherapy Centre, or telephone 0181–202 1439.

# ◆ Index

breasts:
  geranium  107
  pregnancy: recipe  202
breathing, rapid: ylang-ylang
  179
bronchitis: recipes  217, 220
bruises  198
  recipe  233
burners  4, 34
burns: recipe  233
buying essential oils  19–20

cajeput  68–9
camphor  70–1
capillaries, face: recipe  189
car pomanders  39
caraway  72–3
cardamon  74–5
carminative oils  43
carrot seed  76–7
catarrh: recipes  218, 220
cedar of Lebanon  78
cedarwood  12, 78–9
celery  80–1
cellulite
  after birth: recipe  203
  fennel  103
  recipe  233
chamomiles  82–5
chapped hands: recipe  193
chapped lips: recipe  196
chapped skin: recipe  233
cheering, *see* mood lifting
chemical composition, essential
  oils  5

chemicals, synthetic, in
    essential oil preparations
    6
chests, wooden  20
chilblains: recipe  194, 233
childbirth:
  jasmine  114
  recipes after  203–4
children:
  blending for  23
  chamomiles  84
China, aromatics  12–13
cholagogic oils  43
  rose  157
cicatrization  48
cinnamon  86–7
circulatory system  44
  recipes  215–6
citronella  88–9
citrus oils:
  expression  17
  shelf life  21
clarity, lack of  239
clary sage  90–1
Cleopatra  12
clothing, for massage  28
cloudiness:
  avocado oil  8
  essential oils  21–2
clove  92–3
clutter, emotional, mental:
  recipes 239
cold:
  pepper  65
  rosemary  161

*Of further interest...*

# Shirley Price's
# Aromatherapy Workbook
*Understanding essential oils – from plant to bottle*

## Shirley Price

Interest in aromatherapy has burgeoned over the last few years, as people have realized that the vibrant energy of plants, contained in the oils distilled from them, can improve the quality of our lives in many ways.

Going much further than many of the basic guides available today, this book has been written for those who wish to delve deeper into the world of aromatherapy. It includes:

extraction methods for obtaining essential oils
the nature of different carrier oils
therapeutic oils versus perfume oils
plant families and the therapeutic qualities of their essential oils
the chemistry of essential oils
how to use essential oils for health, pleasure and enjoyment.

# Creative Aromatherapy

*Blending and mixing essential oils
and Bach Flower Remedies for health and harmony*

## Christine Wildwood

Aromatherapy is one of the few healing arts which can be
described as creative in an artistic sense. This is because much
of the skill of the adventurous essential oil user lies in his or
her ability to create wonderful aromas by mixing and blending
plant essences, the finest vegetable oils, flower waters, beeswax
and other intriguing substances.
Here Christine Wildwood looks at which oils blend well together,
how our personalities and moods affect these blends, the
different properties and 'notes' of a range of oils, flower remedies
and much more.